Paradigm Shift in Dementia Care

Kenichi Akune, MA

Translated by
Takuro Johnny Hotta and Takahiro Tanaka

CONTENTS

INTRODUCTION

The ultimate care that inspires the "will to live" in people with dementia—this is what I advocated in my book *Dementia Innovation: A Care Method to Create a "Paradise" for Each Individual* (September 2020, President, Inc.).

A "dementia care paradise" is a place where people with dementia can enjoy as much freedom as possible, where their dignity as a person is protected, and their existence, words, and actions are respected. As a means to realize this vision, I wrote *Dementia Innovation* to present a completely new path of dementia care. The book introduces various case studies and experience we have gained at Housenka (nursing and assisted living homes operated by the social welfare corporation Fukusho Fukushikai) as well as the methods we have developed based on the knowledge and know-how we have gained from this experience. Thankfully, we have received many positive responses since its publication.

In particular, we have received numerous comments from the families of those who are residents of Housenka, such as:

"The care provided at Housenka may seem bizarre at first, but after reading the book, I gained a renewed understanding of its meaning and necessity."

"My mother got better once she entered Housenka, and now I know why."

I would like to introduce one letter in particular that we have received from the daughter of one of our residents. In *Dementia Innovation*, we presented the case of Tamae Yamamoto (pseudonym), who would leave her room at night to sleep on the sofa, eat with her hands, or the like. Here is the letter from Mrs. Yamamoto's daughter (excerpted and partially modified).

After reading *Dementia Innovation*, it was clear to me that my mother had received warm and kind care at the facility. She must have been a handful to care for since she left her room at night to sleep on a sofa and ate everything with her hands. The book helped me see that the staff treats the people with dementia in a way that respects their dignity. I'm sure this takes a high amount of insight, patience, and perseverance, and I have nothing but admiration for the staff.

The "Cautionary Aspects of Care that Professionals of Care and Support Must Continue to Keep in Mind" section of the book was very eye-opening. Before reading the book, I had a set of values that I regarded as common sense, and I made sure that my mother's behavior did not deviate from this "norm." After reading this section and reflecting on my past actions, I now understand that this was not only difficult for me, but also for my mother.

Furthermore, I learned that even people with advanced dementia symptoms, like my mother, can still sense how they are being treated. Although we understand the importance of "taking the initiative to respect others," actually doing so can be quite difficult. I thought it was truly wonderful that every staff member of Housenka makes efforts to provide such care. I felt that the foundation of the entire book is "respect," which was very moving.

Such comments and feedback are an encouragement not only to me, but also to all the staff of Housenka. I would like to take this time to thank Mrs. Yamamoto's family and everyone else who sent in their feedback.

Additionally, there were two things about dementia care that I realized as I was writing this book: the importance of "supporting families caring for people with dementia" and "training professionals in dementia care." In reality, there are still many cases in Japan where appropriate dementia care is not provided, and support for families of people with dementia is also insufficient. I could not shake the feeling that this is the reason why the response to my book was so great.

Based on this realization, in October 2021, Housenka established the Green Oasis Meeting, a group meeting for family members who care for those with dementia. This is a place for study and discussion, where people can discuss and empathize with each other about various topics such as understanding dementia, and the anguish and struggles they feel as close family members who support people with dementia. The meeting is held once a month, with some participants attending every meeting while others attending irregularly. It provides a valuable opportunity not only for the families but also for us to communicate with a variety of people and hear their thoughts. The following are some of the comments heard at these meetings.

> "Providing care is difficult because it causes a lot of stress for family members, and there are no opportunities to relieve this stress."
>
> "I feel guilty for being so hard when providing care, and that causes even more stress."
>
> "I get angry because it seems like they are purposely behaving to annoy the people around."
>
> "I subconsciously compare them to when they were not sick."
>
> "It is difficult to determine whether the inability to do something is caused by dementia or they are easily giving up."
>
> "It's frustrating because no matter how many times I tell them, they don't understand."

These opinions and thoughts are only a part of the story; in reality, we cannot ignore the various relationships between parents and children, married couples, and the like when discussing these daily problems.

As I converse with various family members, I realize that family members have only bits and pieces of knowledge and skills regarding dementia, which is understandable. Additionally, since they are family that are close to the person with dementia, they are unable to view the situation objectively, which can lead to negative emotions. I believe this is unavoidable to some extent when close relationships such as family come into play.

I believe that the root of this problem may lie in the fact that families are not asking for enough outside help and are forced to struggle on their own. They are carrying the burden of caregiving alone, or they only build a support system that only involves their immediate family. This self-enclosed form of caregiving results in negative emotions such as, "The problems I'm experiencing are unique and I'm embarrassed to tell people about them," or "I'm afraid people will think I'm not providing proper care." I feel that these negative emotions are the source of suffering for the family members.

Hearing these honest opinions made me keenly aware of the necessity of family support in addition to care for the residents living with dementia themselves. I also strongly felt that conveying our philosophy and methodology of care in a way that families can understand will surely contribute to the development of dementia care professionals.

This is the very reason why I have written this book, which reflects the new knowledge and know-how gained since the publication of my previous book and systematizes and presents the latest care to realize a "dementia care paradise." I hope that this book will enable families and professionals who are engaged in dementia care on a daily basis to provide care with as much serenity as possible.

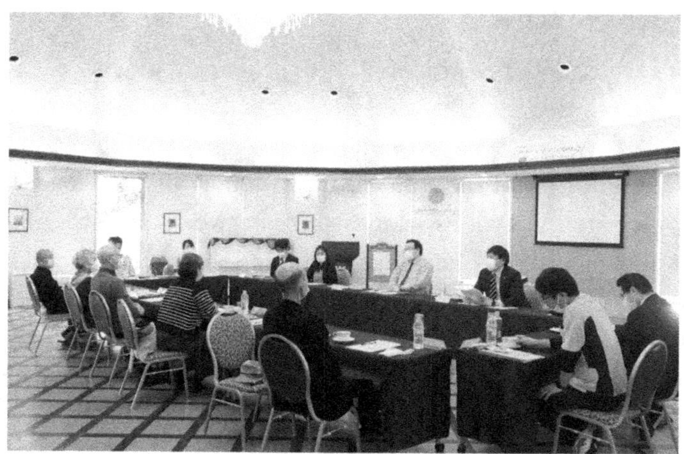

The Green Oasis Meeting, a group meeting for family members who care for those with dementia.

These are some of the serious concerns that family members had before using Housenka. However, with our appropriate care, these residents were able to regain their bright smiles.

Another participant said, "As I provided care, I had almost forgotten how to treat my father with respect, but I was able to reacknowledge what is important after attending the Green Oasis Meeting."

I am proud that we were able to help in situations like these. At the same time, we ourselves are also often surprised to see how the "will to live" in the person with dementia reawakens and flourishes depending on the efforts of our caregivers.

We at Housenka believe that the key to dementia care is to explore ways for people with dementia to live good lives and put it into practice. By helping people with dementia lead independent and peaceful lives according to their circumstances without pain and stress, it also reduces the stress of those who support them, which in turn leads to reestablishing a good relationship with their families.

Rather than viewing issues surrounding dementia as "individual points," that is, correcting the problematic behavior of the person with dementia each time, we must view it through the concept of "dementia complex." In other words, it means we must focus on the whole picture and review the environment surrounding the person with dementia and the life history of the person to create a support system that not only includes long-term care but also medical care, family, and the community. Even if the dementia is irreversible, the important thing is not to give up, but rather accept the situation as is and create a supporting environment that is appropriate to their situation. Only then can we create a wonderful society where everyone, regardless of whether they have dementia or not, can enjoy their lives with vigor and vitality.

In reality, however, we may still be a long way from realizing a dementia care paradise. This is because proper dementia care is not something that can be easily achieved by applying a universal solution. As we will explain later, if there are 100 people with dementia, there will be 100 different care methods. In other words, there is no one solution that applies to all persons with dementia, and appropriate dementia care can only be achieved by pursuing "functional care." Just because a particular approach worked for one person, it does not necessarily mean that it will work for others, and caregivers must continue to work steadily with the person with dementia on a daily basis to determine the appropriate care. In a professional care setting, this must be done with many people at the same time.

As described, there is no one solution for all of our residents at Housenka as well. However, we are able to become aware of many important things on a daily basis, which we use to continue creating dementia care that aims to free people from the anxiety and suffering of dementia. As of 2020, there are around 6.31 million people with dementia in Japan. This number is expected to increase to 11.54 million by 2060. To prepare for this coming age, it is our sincere hope that the dementia care methods introduced in this book will help as many caregivers as possible create "functional care" for as many people with dementia as possible.

CHAPTER 1
ONE IN FIVE WILL SUFFER FROM DEMENTIA

Behaviors That May Be Early Signs of Dementia

The following are symptoms commonly seen in the early stages of dementia. If you notice these behaviors in a family member or acquaintance, it may be early signs of dementia.

1. **Becomes easily irritated or angered.** If someone is becoming irritated for seemingly no reason, it could be a sign that they are not able to grasp the flow of the situation or conversation, leading to anxiety and frustration.

2. **Refuses to bathe.** This could be a sign that complex life activities such as bathing has become a burden. If the person is not bothered by the fact that they have not bathed for days, it may also be a warning.

3. **Many of the same items in the refrigerator.** Some people with dementia forget that they have bought an item and buy it over and over again, or they leave expired items in the refrigerator since they are unable to keep track of expiration dates.

4. **It takes longer to cook familiar dishes, or their cooking tastes different.** Forgetting a recipe for a familiar dish, irregular seasoning, and mistaking sugar and salt are some symptoms seen in people with dementia.

5. **Homes become cluttered.** One of the symptoms of dementia is the inability to clean up and organize. Homes may become filled with garbage.

6. **Stops watching favorite television programs.** This may be caused by loss of motivation or interest, depression, or decrease in concentration or comprehension, which are all early signs.

7. **Behaves inappropriately.** Some types of dementia cause a loss of self-control and lead to inappropriate sexual behavior that would have been unthinkable before suffering from dementia.

8. **Frequently replies irresponsibly.** If a person replies in the same way to any question, or conversations are not making sense, their memory may be affected by dementia.

9. **Makes excuses frequently.** A person may make excuses for many things to hide the fact that they are forgetting or not understanding something.

10. **Change in dietary behavior.** One characteristic of dementia is the tendency to only eat certain foods. There are some cases where the person seems to particularly prefer sweet foods.

These behaviors can be triggered by factors other than dementia, but if more than one of the items listed here apply, it may be an early sign of dementia. We urge you to deepen your understanding of dementia and take appropriate measures. Make sure to visit a physician or hospital that is capable of making a proper diagnosis for an accurate diagnosis.

One in Two Over the Age of 85 Will Have Dementia

Focus on Dementia is Increasing Due to the "Heavily Aging Society"

Japan has one of the world's longest life expectancies. In other words, it is the country facing the most extreme aging problems in the world.

According to the 2022 White Paper on Aging by the Ministry of Health, Labour, and Welfare (MHLW), the percentage of the population aged 65 and older rose from 4.9 percent in 1950 to 12.1 percent in 1990, to 28.6 percent in 2020. It is expected to reach 38.4 percent by 2065.

Among them, the rapid increase in the number of so-called "latter-stage elderly" (those aged 75 and older) is particularly remarkable. Since 2018, the number of latter-stage elderly people have even surpassed that of early-stage elderly people (those aged 65 to 74). This is a condition known as a "super aging society," and is a major social issue, as many people aged 75 and older have declining physical and cognitive abilities.

Statistics show that the number of people requiring long-term care is in fact increasing. Since 2000, when the long-term care insurance system started, the number of those requiring long-term care has increased by approximately 2.6 times as of 2019. This social situation has also led to an increased focus on dementia.

A Common Disease That Can Affect Anyone

In 2012, there were 4.62 million elderly people in Japan with cognitive symptoms. This was 15 percent of the total elderly population, or about one in seven elderly people with dementia. In 2020, this number increased to 6.31 million, or 17.5 percent of the elderly population. This number is further expected to rise to 7.3 million (20.0%) by 2025, meaning that one in five elderly people will have dementia.

Furthermore, it is predicted that by 2060, the number of the elderly population will continue to increase, and the number of people with dementia will reach 11.54 million, accounting for 33.3 percent of the elderly population in Japan (taken from the FY2014 *Summary and Subcommittee Research Report, Study on the Future Population Projection of the Elderly Population with Dementia in Japan*, sponsored by the Health Labour Sciences Research Grant for Special Research). Simply put, this means that one in three elderly people will have dementia. While this data alone is a daunting prospect, we must keep in mind that these figures are for all elderly (those aged 65 and older), and if we narrow it to those aged 75 and older, the percentage of people with dementia will increase even more.

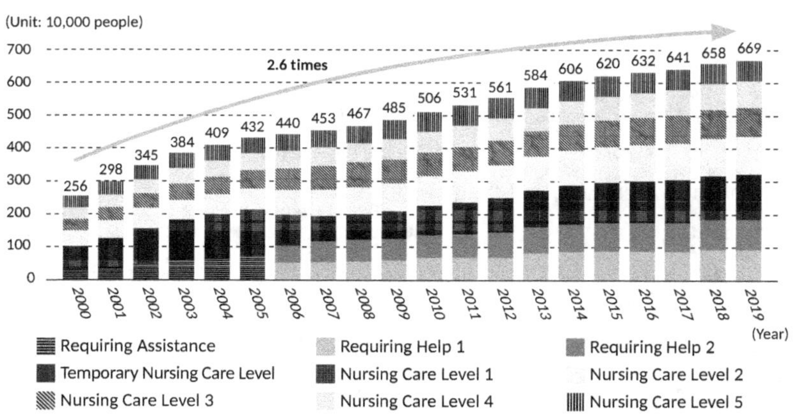

Note: All municipalities have been implementing general nursing care prevention and daily life support projects since FY2017. Due to the Great East Japan Earthquake, the figures for FY2010 do not include the figures for five towns and one village in Fukushima Prefecture.

According to the data published by the Ministry of Health, Labour, and Welfare of Japan (MHLW), only one in 45.5 (2.2 %) people aged 65 to 69 and one in 20 (4.9 %) people aged 70 to 74 have dementia. However, looking further, one in nine (10.9 %) people aged 75 or older, one in four (24.4 %) people aged 80 to 84, and 1.8 in two (55.5 %) people aged 85 or older will be diagnosed with dementia. We can see that the risk of dementia increases with age. Given this data, we can see that the probability of having to live with dementia increases the longer we live. It is actually a common disease that can affect us at any moment. While it would be great if medication were developed to prevent or cure dementia, we must keep in mind that the prevalence of dementia care will continue to increase until that time.

Estimated Number of People with Dementia and Prevalence

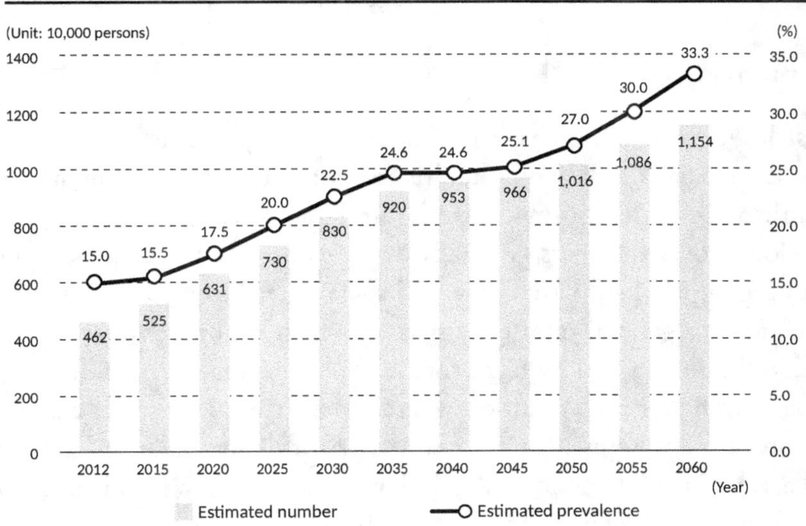

Prevalence of Dementia by Sex and Age Group in 2012 (Calculated from Mathematical Models)

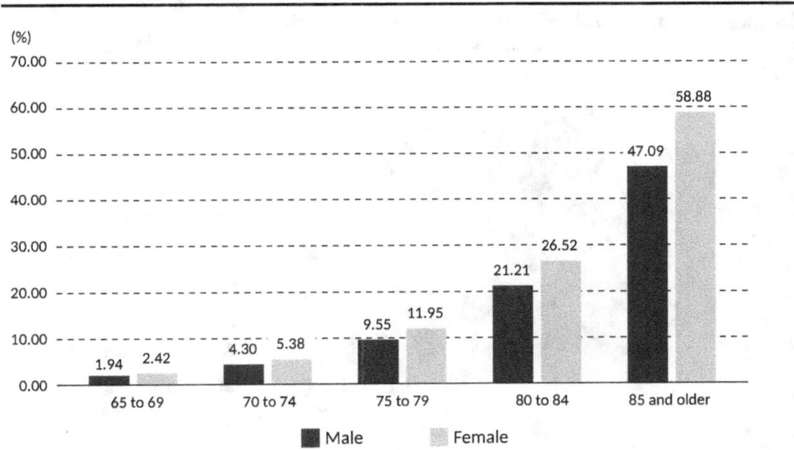

Note: Graph created based on data from the FY2014 Summary and Subcommittee Research Report, Study on the Future Population Projection of the Elderly Population with dementia in Japan, sponsored by the Health Labour Sciences Research Grant for Special Research.

The Four Major Types of Dementia

Dementia Is Not a "Disease" But a "Condition"

First let us review the basics of dementia. Many people tend to think that dementia is a disease, but this is a misconception. Dementia is a condition in which normal memory and cognitive functions that have developed over the years gradually decline due to some acquired cause, resulting in problems in daily life and social interaction. To put it simply, dementia is a general term for a state in which cognitive functions have declined due to a variety of factors. Therefore, dementia is not a single disease; rather, it is a condition where more than 200 diseases can cause symptoms. The four most common types of dementia are Alzheimer's disease, vascular dementia (VaD), dementia with Lewy bodies (DLB), and frontotemporal dementia (FTD). These are sometimes known as the "Big 4 of Dementia." Statistics show that the Big 4 account for a majority of the causes of dementia.

Breakdown of Prevalence by Types of Dementia*:

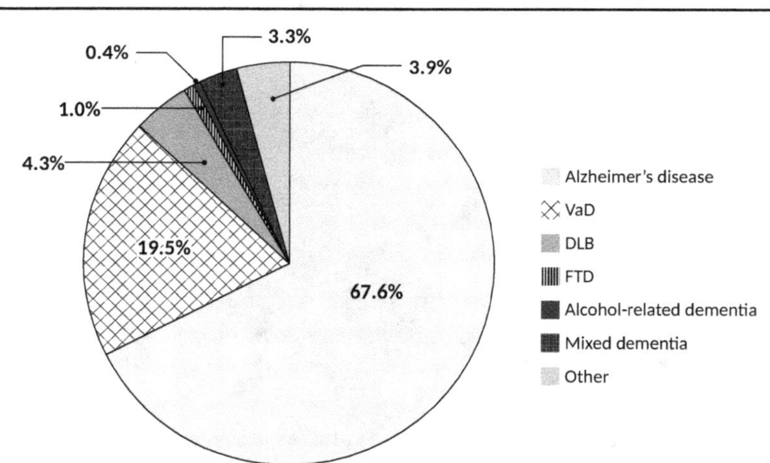

**Data taken from Prevalence of Dementia in Urban Areas and Responses to Impairment of Life Functioning due to Dementia: Comprehensive Research Report FY2011 and 2012 (Takashi Asada, 2013, sponsored by the Health Labour Sciences Research Grant for General Dementia Control Research).*

Breakdown of prevalence by types of dementia:

(1) Alzheimer's disease: 67.6 %
(2) VaD: 19.5 %
(3) DLB: 4.3 %
(4) FTD: 1.0 %
(5) Alcohol-related dementia: 0.4 %
(6) Mixed dementia: 3.3 %
(7) Other: 3.9 %

Types (1), (3), and (4) are classified as neurodegenerative diseases, (2) as cerebrovascular diseases, (6) as a mixture of the above two types, and (5) as substance-related diseases. In addition, endocrine diseases that cause hypothyroidism, neoplastic diseases such as normal pressure hydrocephalus, infectious diseases such as Creutzfeldt-Jakob disease and those that cause diseases such as encephalitis and AIDS can also cause dementia, as can drugs, hypoxemia from respiratory diseases, psychiatric diseases such as depression, and long periods of undernutrition.

While some of these cognitive symptoms may improve with treatment of the disease, organic changes in the brain are generally considered irreversible. In other words, while there may be some improvement in cognitive function, recovering to the same state as before contracting the disease is unlikely. This is another important point when trying to understand dementia.

Now let's take a look at the specific causes, common symptoms, and other details about the Big 4 of dementia.

Alzheimer's Disease: A Gradual Atrophy of the Brain

Alzheimer's disease is by far the most common type of dementia.

Amyloid beta and tau proteins can accumulate in the brain over a period of more than a decade, which destroys cerebral nerve cells and leads to atrophy of the brain. It usually begins by affecting the hippocampus, the part of the brain responsible for memory, and eventually the entire cerebrum is affected.

While there are obviously individual differences, the transition of symptoms can generally be broadly divided into early, middle, and late stages. The disease usually progresses over a span of about ten years.

In the early (mild) stage, the person may experience strong stress and symptoms of depression due to anxiety and agitation stemming from their declining memory. At this stage, the person often notices that something is wrong, but family members and others are often unaware of the onset of the disease. Specific symptoms include memory impairment, in which the person forgets conversations and repeatedly says or asks the same thing; delusions of theft, in which the person thinks items such as wallets and bankbooks that they misplaced were stolen; and disorientation, in which the day of the month, day of the week, or time of day becomes vague for the person. However, in the early stages, many people can cover up their impairment and pretend nothing is wrong. Another symptom is executive dysfunctions, such as loss of interest, apathy, inability to perform familiar household chores and routine tasks, and inability to use familiar equipment.

In the middle stage (moderate), physical functions are still maintained but cognitive decline becomes more noticeable. Cognitive symptoms include a severe impairment in memory, judgment, comprehension, and orientation while behavioral and psychological symptoms of dementia (BPSD) become more common. For example, the person with dementia may put dangerous or dirty things in their mouth due to impaired judgment. Other symptoms include the inability to choose clothing appropriate for the season; wandering around due to confusion about the current time, era, or place; inability to reach a destination; inability to return home; and wearing different footwear on each foot when going out. Other symptoms to keep in mind are aphasia, in which the person loses the ability to understand the meaning of words or to speak properly, and apraxia, in which the person loses the ability to clean up, eat, or get dressed independently. The person may defecate in places other than a toilet, or touch feces and touch clothes, objects, or their own face or body without washing their hands. This is a very difficult time for both the person with dementia and the caregiver, as the person becomes increasingly confused due to anxiety and fear.

In the late (severe) stage, disorientation that impairs perception of the current time, season, and location becomes more common. The person may also have trouble recognizing people and may not be able to recognize family members or may not recognize their own face in a mirror. At this stage, motor functions are also affected. The person may lose the ability to walk, stand or sit up, eat by themselves, or swallow food properly. Even worse, they may become bedridden. They may also become less responsive or unresponsive when spoken to and may also lose facial expressions. Statistics show that women are more likely than men to be affected by this disease.

Vascular Dementia: Causes of Varying Levels of Cognitive Symptoms and Emotional Incontinence

Vascular dementia (VaD) is a general term for cognitive symptoms that appear as a result of a stroke caused by cerebral infarction or cerebral hemorrhage. Cerebral infarctions are said to be the most common cause of VaD.

Cerebral infarction can be broadly classified into two types: a type in which a large blood vessel becomes clogged and causes rapid change, and a type in which small, thin blood vessels become clogged and the condition progresses gradually. The latter includes multiple lacunar infarct (multiple small strokes) and Binswanger's disease, both of which are difficult to recognize, and even when cognitive symptoms appear, they may be assumed to be part of aging. Although symptoms and the degree of symptoms that appear vary on factors such as whether the person had a cerebral infarction or cerebral hemorrhage and individual differences, in general, executive dysfunction is more prominent than memory impairment such as forgetfulness. The symptoms also differ depending on which part of the brain was damaged. Damage to the parietal lobe causes disorientation and apraxia, while damage to the frontal lobe, which controls emotional functions, causes depression. Attention span may also decrease, which can cause symptoms such as neglecting other tasks to focus on one task, difficulty doing two tasks at once, difficulty maintaining concentration, and becoming easily distracted.

Other common symptoms include:

- Varying levels of cognitive symptoms: Since only parts of the brain are damaged, the person may show a mixture of impaired and normal abilities. For example, memory impairment may be mild, but executive function may be impaired, or forgetfulness may be present, but judgment may be unaffected. General motivation may also fluctuate.

- Emotional incontinence: The person may experience difficulty controlling their emotions. They may suddenly become angry, laugh, or cry, or have sudden mood swings. They may cry when casually greeted, or smile but actually be in a bad mood. Their emotions may be bursting one moment then suddenly become emotionless the next.

- Fluctuations: The person's ability, motivation and emotional stability fluctuates during the course of a day. Since the person may be aware at times that they have memory impairment and are losing the ability to do many tasks, caregivers must be careful since passing remarks may damage the person's self-esteem.

- Motor dysfunction: This includes motor paralysis of limbs, gait disorder caused by numbness and other sensory paralysis, dysphagia, dysuria, and speech disorders.

- Nocturnal delirium: This refers to the condition in which disorientation (a temporary loss of perception of time and location), or mental disturbances such as the sudden loss of ability to think, occur during the night. It is most often seen in elders and manifests itself at night with symptoms such as loss of coherence, loss of awareness of time and location, memory loss, waking up at night, hallucinations, and delusions. Statistics show that men are more likely to be affected by this disease.

Dementia with Lewy Bodies: Causes Hallucinations and Delusions

Cognitive symptoms are caused when special proteins called Lewy bodies accumulate in the cerebral cortex and brainstem, which destroys nerve cells. One characteristic of DLB is that hallucinations and delusions are common in the early stages of the disease. Visual hallucinations seem to be the most common type of hallucination, and the person complains of seeing children, animals, insects, and people who have already died. To the person, the hallucination they are experiencing seems very real, which may frighten them.

Symptoms of delusions include behaviors such as trying to commute to a workplace they no longer work at, acting as if they are in wartime, and trying to go home even though they are already at home. The person will also have major fluctuations in mood and awareness, even within a short period of time. There are also severe fluctuations from day to day, which also extends to cognitive functions. The buildup of Lewy bodies in the brain stem can also lead to symptoms of Parkinson's. This can cause muscle stiffness, postural instability, slowness of movements, and tremors, which can lead to gait disturbance or hypomimia, which is a loss of facial expression. Other characteristic symptoms of DLB include abnormal behavior such as sleep-talking loudly or sleepwalking, and constipation, fatigue, decreased appetite, urination problems, sweating disorders, low blood pressure, and the like caused by autonomic nervous system dysfunction.

Depression is also common in the early stages, and mood swings and lethargy are often observed. Since memory impairment and forgetfulness do not commonly appear as a symptom, the person may be misdiagnosed as having depression or other mental disorders. As the condition progresses, memory impairment and forgetfulness occur, and the person's ability to make judgments and understand things deteriorates, gradually interfering with daily life. Men are twice as likely as women to develop the disease.

Frontotemporal Dementia: Causes Personality Changes and Behavioral/Language Disorders

Frontotemporal dementia (FTD) is a brain atrophy caused by a gradual decrease in nerve cells due to a buildup of tau and other proteins in the frontal lobes—which control social skills, personality, reason, and language—and in the temporal lobes—which control language comprehension, memory, and voice recognition. It is a form of frontotemporal lobar degeneration (FTLD). FTLD is broadly classified into three types: (1) FTD; (2) semantic dementia, which affects semantic memory and causes a person to lose the ability to understand, read, or write words or recognize the faces of family members and other close people; and (3) progressive nonfluent aphasia (PNFA), which causes speech disorders such as losing the ability to make grammatically-correct sentences, pronounce words correctly, speak smoothly, or carry out conversations at a normal pace.

Of those diagnosed with FTD, behavioral variant frontotemporal dementia (BvFTD; previously known as Pick's disease), characterized by the spherical inclusion bodies called Pick bodies found in the neurons of the brain, is said to account for half of all cases. BvFTD often develops in early life (age 40 to 60), and it is rare for it to develop in people older than age 70. In the early stages of the disease, symptoms usually associated with dementia, such as forgetfulness and memory loss are not seen, so the person and those around may not be able to recognize the onset of the disease. Keep in mind that atrophy of the frontal and temporal lobes, which cause personality and behavioral changes, may occur even when Pick bodies are not present.

The following are other common symptoms:

- Loss of motivation: This appears as symptoms such as stopping favorite activities such as watching TV and reading the newspaper, losing interest in things, and becoming lazy. The person may talk less or lose their expressive abilities, resulting in simpler conversations such as replying irresponsibly or giving the same answer to all questions.

- Understanding of language decreases: This appears as symptoms such as failing to recall the meaning of words or names, misreading words, or losing the ability to recognize letters.

- Loss of emotions: This appears as symptoms such as diminished interest in others and losing the ability to empathize with others or read emotions. Even while with other people, they may suddenly leave if they lose interest. They will also be less expressive of their emotions.

- Loss of social skills: The disease will cause the person to act more instinctively, and impulsive behavior that is hard to control—such as a lack of consideration for their surroundings, acting impolitely without discretion, or shouting or becoming violent when they lose their temper—will increase. In some cases, the person will lose their moral and ethical values, causing them to shoplift, steal, dine and dash, or urinate in public. These behaviors are not done with malicious intent, rather they are purely acting on instinct. Many people will continue to behave the same way even after they are warned, so caregivers must get creative to control the behavior. Another common symptom is a loss of care regarding personal appearance.

- Change in dietary behavior: This appears as symptoms such as an increased appetite, only eating a particular dish, and consuming excessive amounts of sugar, sweets, juices, and other sweet foods. They may swallow without chewing enough, causing them to eat at a faster pace.

- Routine behavior: Patterned, routine, behavior, such as performing a certain action at a certain time each day as if following a timetable, will be prevalent. They may also perform the same behavior, such as clapping their hands, repeatedly.

- Easily affected by environmental stimuli: The person will seem to be more sensitive to visual and audio information. This appears as symptoms such as repeating what someone said repetitively, subconsciously imitating the action of others, reading words they see out loud, or using any object that they see without permission.

- Inappropriate sexual behavior: This is caused by a loss of self-control. It appears as symptoms such as indecent exposure, improper sexual language and behavior, molestation, and obsession with pornographic videos and services. In many cases, these actions lead to the police getting involved. There have also been cases where the person is restless and has difficulty maintaining focus.

As the disease progresses, behavioral symptoms are suppressed due to a further loss of motivation, and appetite decreases as well. In many cases, the person becomes bedridden within six to nine years after the onset of the disease. The onset of the disease often occurs at an early elderly age, and it affects men and women equally.

Mixed Dementia: Onset of Multiple Dementias

Sometimes more than one of the previously described types of dementia or other types may develop, and this is called mixed dementia.

While the most common is a combination of Alzheimer's disease and VaD, there have been cases of Alzheimer's disease combined with DLB or the like. Since the risk of developing dementia increases as people get older, mixed dementia is inevitably more prevalent as the age group advances.

As described above, there are a variety of illnesses that can cause the Big 4 of dementia and other types. The most important factor in responding appropriately is to understand the current situation correctly, and the first step is to get a proper diagnosis. Rather than assuming that dementia cannot be cured and giving up, it is important to determine the disease or other factor that is causing the dementia. There have been cases where treating the disease have led to an improvement in cognitive symptoms.

Mild Cognitive Impairment: An Early Indicator of Dementia with Symptoms Such As Memory Loss

Mild cognitive impairment (MCI) is a condition in which cognitive functions are slightly impaired but do not meet the criteria to be diagnosed as dementia. Although the condition does not interfere with activities of daily living (ADL) significantly, a person with MCI cannot be classified as normal. It can be said as an area between normal aging and dementia and may be an early indicator of dementia.

To be diagnosed as MCI, a person must meet the following criteria**:

- Memory impairment that cannot be explained solely by the effects of normal aging or educational background

- Complains of memory loss by the person themselves or a family member

- General cognitive function is within the normal range

- Can independently conduct activities of daily living

- The person is not diagnosed with dementia

** Taken from *e-Health Net*, a publicly-accessible health information website for the prevention of lifestyle-related diseases by MHLW.

In short, the person has memory impairment and is aware of their forgetfulness, but there is no obvious impairment in other cognitive abilities, and there is little to no impact on daily life.

While some people recover from MCI, it is estimated that 10 to 15 percent of people with MCI will transition to dementia annually, which is why it is considered an early indicator of dementia.

The Difference Between Age-Related Forgetfulness and Dementia

We are often asked what the difference is between age-related forgetfulness and dementia. The biggest indicator is the difference between forgetting an entire experience (dementia) or only a part of it (age-related).

For a person with dementia, they may not even know that they are forgetting because the memory of an experience or specific details like the date has disappeared. On the other hand, for age-related forgetfulness, the person is only partial forgetting; they are aware that they are forgetting and will remember when given hints about the event or the like.

For example, let's say a person has promised to get dinner with a friend. If the person has dementia, they may completely forget that they made plans. When the friend calls to remind them of the plan, the person with dementia may become angry and claim that they did not make plans, or they may become suspicious of the friend and claim no responsibility for their actions. In some cases, the person may tell incoherent stories or make peculiar excuses.

On the other hand, in the case of age-related forgetfulness, the person will remember the plan when the friend calls and apologize since they know that they were wrong. They can act accordingly, such as by rushing to meet up with the friend or rescheduling. In addition to forgetfulness, dementia is characterized by a decline in such life functions and judgment.

In recent years, focus has been increasing on early onset dementia, which is defined as the development of Alzheimer's disease or other types of dementia before the age of 65.

In 2017 to 2019, the number of those aged 18 to 64 with early onset dementia was estimated to be 35,700, which is 5.1 per 10,000 persons between age 18 to 64. The average age of onset is 54.4. In cases where the person's career is on the rise when the disease strikes, they may become self-destructive or develop depression, and the support of family members is essential (for more detail, refer to *Prevalence and Number of Patients with Early Onset Dementia in Japan*, July 2020, by the Tokyo Metropolitan Geriatric Hospital and Institute of Gerontology).

Cognitive Symptoms and Behavioral and Psychological Symptoms of Dementia

The Two Types of Dementia Symptoms

To properly understand dementia, it is also important to know that the symptoms of dementia can be divided into two main types. One is the "cognitive symptoms" directly caused by changes to the brain, and the other is the "Behavioral and Psychological Symptoms of Dementia (BPSD)," which are symptoms that accompany the cognitive symptoms.

The following is a brief description of symptoms divided by type.

Behavioral and psychological symptoms of dementia (BPSD)

Behavioral symptoms	Cognitive symptoms	Psychological symptoms
Wandering	Memory impairment	Anxiety
Collecting items	Disorientation	Depression
Verbal and physical violence	Decrease in comprehension and judgment	Apathy, indifferent
Abnormal eating habits	Executive dysfunction	Does not talk
Insomnia, nocturnal	Aphasia	Delusions (paranoia)
Resists care	Apraxia	Visual and auditory hallucinations
Slowness of movement	Agnosia	Other
Short temper/agitated	Other	
Inappropriate sexual behavior		
Other		

Irritable

Cognitive Symptoms

Cognitive symptoms such as memory impairment and disorientation become apparent first.

- **Memory impairment:** First, recent memory (memory of learning and experiences from the last few minutes to days) begins to be impaired, making it difficult to remember the most recent events. As symptoms progress, the impairment spreads to remote memory (memories of decades worth of experiences) and immediate memory (memories of a few seconds).

- **Disorientation:** This refers to a condition in which a person becomes unable to recognize the current date, day of the week, season, location, or familiar person. In general, the person first loses track of the time, such as the day of the week, followed by location, and then loses the ability to distinguish between people.

- **Difficulty understanding:** The person may have difficulty understanding the meaning or details of something they see, have discrepancies between their thoughts or words and their actual actions, or have difficulty engaging in complex conversations or operating equipment.

- **Impaired judgment:** The person may lose moral and ethical values, and act against the law or social rules, such as shoplifting or dining and dashing, which may lead to legal action or accidents.

- **Executive dysfunction:** Decreased memory, reasoning, concentration, attention, planning, judgment, and the like results in the inability to efficiently perform household chores or follow a plan when working.

- **Aphasia:** Damage to the language center of the brain results in symptoms such as the inability to speak well, read or write, or understand the meaning of questions.

- **Apraxia:** A person will have difficulty performing activities of daily living despite the absence of paralysis or abnormal physical functions. They will have difficulties buttoning a jacket or using eating utensils.

- **Agnosia:** Although vision, hearing, and the sense of touch are not impaired, the person will have difficulties understanding the meaning or the distance and location of what they see.

Behavioral and Psychological Symptoms of Dementia (BPSD)

Peripheral symptoms that accompany the cognitive symptoms are divided into "behavioral symptoms" and "psychological symptoms."

Psychological Symptoms:

- **Delusions:** This is a condition in which a person has strong false beliefs in things that are not real. Delusions of theft are particularly common. They also often become paranoid.

- **Hallucinations:** This is the condition in which a person perceives something that does not exist as real. It can affect any sense, causing visual, auditory, tactile, and olfactory hallucinations.

- **Illusions:** This is the condition in which a person perceives something as something different from what it actually is. The person may look at a piece of rope and think it is a bug or mishear words such as "spoon" as, for example, "soap" or "soup."

- **Nocturnal delirium:** This is the condition in which minor mental disturbances such as disorientation, delusions, hallucinations, and illusions occur only at night.

- **Emotional incontinence:** This is the condition in which a person loses emotional control, leading to sudden bursts of laughter, crying, or anger over trivial matters.

- **Anxiety and depression:** A decline in cognitive abilities can cause symptoms such as increased anxiety, depression, decreased motivation, and loss of appetite.

- **Apathy:** This is the condition in which a person quits hobbies such as cooking, declines social gatherings even if they used to be very sociable, or loses interest in everything.

- **Personality change:** The person becomes less considerate of others and acts in a self-centered manner or acts inappropriately due to an inability to judge right from wrong.

- **Irritable:** The person becomes more irritable because the change in condition limits their actions and builds up anxiety.

Behavioral Symptoms:

- **Wandering:** The person wanders both inside and outside the house and may not be able to return once they leave the house.

- **Routine strolls:** The person walks a set course at a set time each day. In general, they will return home on their own.

- **Abusive language:** The person may curse or say hurtful words in a harsh tone.

- **Violence:** The person may throw and break things, kick, and punch others, and sometimes try to use blades.

- **Agitated:** A highly emotional state in which the person is unable to control their emotions well.

- **Talking to self:** The person may be talking to themselves but act as if they are having a conversation. They may smirk profoundly even when nothing interesting is going on.

- **Short temper:** The person suddenly becomes angry over trivial matters as if their personality has changed, or a previously mild-mannered person becomes short-tempered.

- **Resists care:** This is the condition in which a person refuses to accept care from caregivers. They may refuse in a variety of situations, such as refusal to take a bath or refusal to take medications.

- **Inappropriate sexual behavior:** Behaviors such as talking to strangers of the opposite sex in public places, indecent exposure, masturbation, and buying large amounts of pornographic videos or watching them in public are observed.

- **Desire to return home:** The person may have a strong desire to return home not only while outdoors, but also when they are already at home. They may try to leave the house or become impatient.

- **Abnormal eating habits:** The person may only eat what they like or only eat certain foods, which prevents them from eating a well-balanced diet. They may also put non-edible items in their mouths or have low fluid intake.

- **Improper urination and defecation:** The person may urinate or defecate in improper places (such as hallways and dining rooms) for reasons such as forgetting the location of bathrooms.

- **Sleep disorders:** The person's sleep may be shallow, causing them to wake up quickly after sleeping and move around at night, resulting in a disturbance of their sleep rhythm. It is not uncommon for the day and nights to be reversed for those with dementia.

- **Smearing:** The person may not wipe properly after defecating, or smear feces on beds or tables.

- **Plays with food:** The person may mix all the food in front of them and stir it with utensils or their hands.

Symptoms are Different For All, Hence the Need for Functional Care

It is important to note that there is no set rule regarding which of the above symptoms will appear. Symptoms that appear and their degree may be different depending on the person, even for the same type of dementia.

BPSD are caused by a combination of "cognitive symptoms" (symptoms brought on by the disease), "personal experience of thoughts, culture, and life history," and "the person's physical functions." Therefore, each case of dementia will result in a different *condition*. In fact, I have dealt with many people with dementia throughout my career, and the symptoms they show and the reality they see are very different from one another. This means that there is no universal solution for dementia care, and it requires a tailored response for each individual.

Factors of BPSD

Cognitive symptoms

||

Symptoms brought on by the disease

✕

[Personal experience of thoughts × culture × life history]

✕

Physical functions

Social Impact of the Rise In Dementia

Measures Against Dementia Leads to an Increase in Social Costs

An increase in the number of people with dementia will have a variety of social impacts. In particular, the following four are expected to have major impacts.

    (1) Increase in social costs
    (2) Increase in the number of people quitting jobs to provide care
    (3) Increase in the number of missing persons
    (4) Expansion of market for related products and services

The social cost related to dementia was estimated at 14.5 trillion yen as of 2014. The breakdown is approximately 6.4 trillion yen for long-term care, 1.9 trillion yen for medical care, and 6.2 trillion yen for informal care by family members and the like. In other words, the costs of long-term care and informal care account for a larger share of the social costs than medical costs.

In the above study, the annual cost of informal care per person requiring long-term care was estimated to be 382.1 million yen per year, based on an average of 24.97 hours of informal care per person per week. However, since the study only included those who receive long-term care services, and since the estimate did not consider the indirect time required for caregivers such as looking after the person with dementia (judging from the fact that the amount of time allocated to informal care only comes out to 3.56 hours per day), the estimated cost does not reflect all costs associated with informal care. The reality of informal care costs should be much higher when including the substantial number of people caring for those with dementia at home.

Of further concern is that the number of people with dementia is expected to increase from 5.25 million in 2015 to 7.3 million in 2025, a 1.4-fold increase over a decade. In conjunction with this increase, social costs are also estimated to swell to 19.5 trillion yen. In addition, looking at further estimates of the increase in the people with dementia and social costs, it is predicted that in 2045 there will be 9.66 million people with dementia and social costs will be 22.5 trillion yen, increasing to 11.54 million people and 24.3 trillion yen by 2060 (data excerpted from the FY2014 *Summary and Subcommittee Research Report: Study on the Economic Impact of Dementia in Japan*, sponsored by the Health Labour Sciences Research Grant for General Dementia Control Research [partially revised]). Given the fact that there are also other hidden costs, it is an alarming fact that the social costs of dementia are quite enormous, especially the costs associated with care, such as long-term care costs and informal care costs.

Factors of BPSD

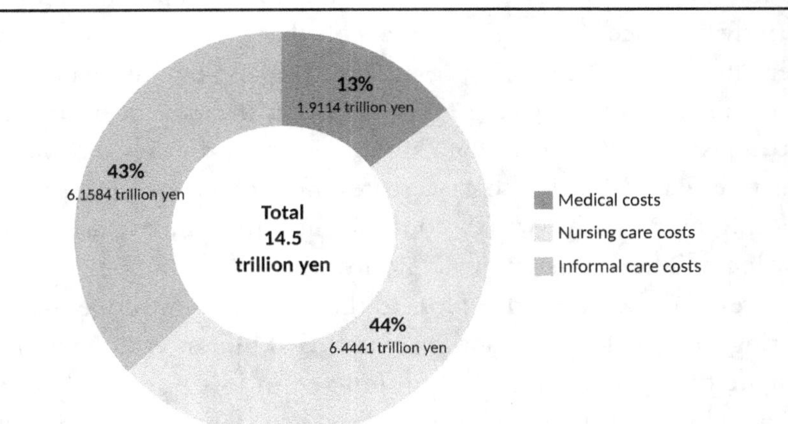

Source: Graph created based on the FY2014 Summary and Subcommittee Research Report, Study on the Economic Impact of dementia in Japan, sponsored by the Health Labour Sciences Research Grant for General dementia Control Research.

In light of these issues, serious consideration should be given to how resources should be allocated to reduce the burden on caregivers and to improve the quality of life and dignity of people with dementia and their families. Cost-effectiveness studies will be required to examine not only the social costs themselves, but also whether these costs are leading to effective care.

We truly believe that providing effective care as possible through Housenka's care methods will contribute to solving these social issues surrounding dementia. Expensive care that only overwhelms both the person with dementia and the caregiver will not lead to happiness for anyone, nor is it cost-effective. Nothing would make us happier than if our methods can make even a small contribution to reducing or improving social costs.

Employees Quitting to Provide Care Is a Major Blow to Companies

The second impact of dementia on society is the increase in the number of people quitting jobs to provide care. The number of people quitting to provide care, which was 49,000 in 2007, increased to 92,000 by 2017, a two-fold increase in only ten years. Although the number has remained relatively flat since 2013, it is quite possible that this number will increase given the future increase in the number of people with dementia (as based on *Employment Trend Survey*, MHLW). The increase in employees quitting is a major blow to companies. Not only do they lose valuable human resources, but it also exacerbates the problem of labor shortages affecting many fields, which could eventually lead to an economic slowdown. The Ministry of Economy, Trade, and Industry (METI) estimates that the value-added loss to the entire economy due to people quitting to provide care is approximately 650 billion yen, including an estimate of approximately 270 billion yen in lost potentially-earned individual income, based on average wages and other factors as well as the total impact on the added value generated by companies and the like. (For more detail, please refer to *Structural Changes in the Economy and Society by 2050 and Policy Issues*, METI, September 2018).

The data indicate that dementia and associated care will not only affect social security costs, but also the labor force, which is the source of social security funds, and in turn, deliver a major blow to companies. If we do not consider this fact to improve the environment for caregivers, we will end up in a vicious cycle in which the increase in the number of people requiring long-term care due to the aging of the population will lead to an increase in the number of people leaving the workforce, resulting in a decrease in social security budgets and further worsening the long-term care environment. Highly effective dementia care that brings happiness to both the person with dementia and the caregivers is necessary to break this negative cycle.

Wandering Leads to Missing Persons

The third impact is the increase in missing persons. According to an announcement by the National Police Agency of Japan in June 2022, the number of cases of people with dementia or those suspected of having dementia going missing due to wandering or other reasons has been increasing. In 2021, 17,636 cases were reported, the highest number since 2012, when the statistics were first collected. While most of those people were located within a week, 236 people remain missing. Additionally, of those who have been reported missing in the past, 450 people were found dead on the streets in 2021. In some cases, the person who was wandering ended up in a traffic accident or was found in unpopulated areas such as in the mountains.

Sometimes, a person with dementia will escape a nursing home without permission. This is not uncommon and happens in many facilities nationwide. We have experienced a few cases at Housenka but fortunately, so far it has not led to serious problems, and all residents were returned safely. While we were lucky that nothing more serious happened, this is an issue that must be discussed thoroughly to prevent it from happening at all. Since escapes occur even in nursing homes that have ample security measures and under the watchful eye of multiple staff members, it is easy to conclude that it is a lot more common for a person to wander out of their own homes, where the number of caregivers is limited. Just because the number of missing persons due to dementia is increasing, we believe it is shortsighted to think of this behavior as tough to handle or a nuisance. It may have a specific cause such as delusions and hallucinations. Or the person with dementia may simply be trying to fulfill their desires such as wanting to go for a walk, have a change of scenery, or go shopping.

Some nursing homes may think that the proper measures are focused solely on safety and therefore will trap residents by completely locking all entrances and preventing windows from opening. However, this would deprive residents of their dignity as human beings and cause them further stress. Given this reality, there is an urgent need to establish a system in which society as a whole can better look after those with dementia.

Expansion of Dementia-Related Markets

On the other hand, not all social impacts are negative. There is also the growing market for products and services related to dementia. For example, iTSUMO by Urbantech is a GPS device for those who wander and try to escape facilities. It can ensure the safety of a person with dementia while still allowing them freedom. The GPS device is attached to the person's shoe, and it will monitor them when they leave the house or facility.

As digital transformation progresses in society, the long-term care field must also stop relying only on staffing (supported by human hands) and adapt to using ICT and IoT to provide care. By utilizing digital devices, it will become easier to build a system where society or the community as a whole watch over and support people with dementia. This in turn will lead to the realization of care that balances freedom and safety. The development of drugs to reverse or treat dementia is also progressing worldwide (as will be discussed later). As we can see, the research and development related to dementia also has many economic benefits.

Do Not Think of Dementia as Embarrassing

As stated above, the increase in the number of people with dementia has had a significant impact on society, and this impact is expected to grow even further in the future. In an age when anyone can develop dementia, the concept of "living with dementia" is required in society. As nuclear family households have become the norm, the number of households with only elderly members is increasing. Combined with the increase in average lifespan, the result has been an increase in "elder-on-elder care," where the elder is forced to provide care for another elder, and "dementia-on-dementia care," where those with dementia are forced to provide care for others with dementia. Furthermore, many elderly people who require nursing care or who have dementia are forced to live alone. For some family members, care for a loved one at home—even if the caregiver is in good health—the caregiving takes up so much time and energy that employment and/or schoolwork are neglected. Many caregivers become so overwhelmed that they must bear just trying to make it through the day. We can assume that the harsh reality of providing care leads to the increase in the number of missing persons with dementia, and perhaps tragedies such as abuse and murder by caregivers.

Appropriate dementia care cannot be completed simply through family love or "self-responsibility." Rather than leaving the responsibility of care to the family or a single caregiver alone, it is necessary to build a system to support care more broadly in society. To this end, it is essential that more people become aware of the current situation and build a system to extend a helping hand.

Although within the confines of our local community, we at Housenka also cooperate with community-wide efforts to watch over people with dementia, such as the dementia and Disability Wandering SOS Mail for Toyonaka City, Osaka, and the Minoh Missing Person SOS Net in Minoh City, Osaka. In the event that we receive a report from the police or local government concerning a missing person, we will assist in the search for the missing person while making rounds in the community to pick up and drop off facility users.

Throughout Japan, MHLW also trains "dementia supporters," who have the correct knowledge and understanding of dementia and support people with dementia and their families in the community. A society where each person can do one or more simple things to help will lead to communities where people with dementia will be able to live with peace of mind. We truly hope that such activities will spread further, and that our society will become one in which people with dementia can live without worries.

As dementia is becoming a common disease, we believe that people must become more aware of dementia and people with dementia. While it is understandable that it is difficult to be interested in dementia if it does not concern us, if we do not have the proper knowledge when we or a family member develops dementia, we will have to rush to gather information about dementia and long-term care, making it difficult to understand or respond appropriately.

The reality is that Japan's life expectancy is long and the number of those requiring long-term care is increasing, so it is necessary for everyone to raise awareness and abandon stereotypical ideas that dementia is something to be ashamed of or to hide. Start by acquiring knowledge about measures and care in advance to prepare for any situation. This may ultimately help you and your family, raise the level of dementia literacy, and save family members providing care from loneliness.

Will Dementia Become Reversible? The Future of Treatment

Development of Drugs to Reverse or Treat Dementia and New Care Methods are Progressing

According to the *Global Status Report on the Public Health Response to Dementia Executive Summary* published by the World Health Organization (WHO) in 2021, 55.2 million people around the world had dementia in 2019, and 1.6 million people died from the disease in the same year. dementia is the seventh leading cause of death on a global scale. The number of people with dementia continues to increase and is projected to reach 78 million by 2030 and 139 million by 2050. This shows that dementia is an issue that is not unique to Japan but rather, a global issue.

To tackle this issue, nations and companies are fiercely competing with each other to develop drugs to prevent, treat, or reverse dementia. In 1999, Aricept—the world's first drug that improves cognitive function—was approved for use in Japan (it was approved in the U.S.A. in 1996). Since then, many drugs for Alzheimer's disease have been developed, but only a few have been proven effective. Pharmaceutical companies Eisai Co., Ltd. (Japan) and Biogen Inc. (U.S.) applied to the U.S. Food and Drug Administration (FDA) in July 2020 for approval of Aducanumab—a potential treatment for Alzheimer' disease—but questions were raised about the clinical trial process during the approval review. It was granted conditional approval in June 2021. In Japan, an application for approval was submitted to MHLW in December 2020, but the application was declined in December 2021 and is still under review.

In January 2023, the FDA confirmed the efficacy of Lecanemab—a new Alzheimer's disease drug also developed by Eisai Co., Ltd. (Japan) and Biogen Inc. (U.S.)—during the final stages of development and granted it accelerated approval. The companies are working to get it fully approved. A new drug application was also filed in Japan in January 2023.

Other Alzheimer's disease drugs such as Donanemab, developed by Eli Lilly and Company (U.S.), and Gantenerumab, developed by F. Hoffmann-La Roche AG (Switzerland), are currently undergoing clinical trials. The hope is that drugs to treat or prevent dementia will be available in the future.

In addition to drugs, light therapy and ultrasound therapy are also being developed as new treatment options. Not only is the development of these non-drug options desired by people with dementia and their families, but it is also expected to have a positive economic impact.

New testing methods that use technology to diagnose dementia from various perspectives, such AI-based diagnostic support systems for physicians, tests to determine the accumulation of amyloid beta in the brain only using a small amount of blood, and data analysis of words uttered by a person to determine extent of dementia, are also being approved and introduced in the field.

Research on dementia care is also being conducted worldwide, and the accumulation of knowledge is accelerating. For example, *The 36-Hour Day* (Nancy L. Mace, MA and Peter V. Rabins, MD, MPH, Johns Hopkins University Press) compiles information on the best dementia care practices and cutting-edge dementia research. It was first published in the U.S. in 1981 and revised editions with updated information have been published to date. Currently translated into more than ten languages, it is widely read by families of people with dementia as well as professionals in the medical and long-term care fields. The Japanese translation of *The 36-Hour Day,* (6th edition, translated by

Takahiro Tanaka, Representative Director of SF Housenka and CEO of Lighthouse Health Inc., through Cross Media Publishing) will be published in fall 2023.

Development of new dementia care is also progressing in Denmark, considered the leading welfare state, and other countries such as Sweden, the Netherlands, France, and the U.S. The Positive Health concept, which originated in the Netherlands, is based on the idea that "health" is the ability to utilize various strengths and live positively in life despite illness or disability, and we feel that this concept has many things in common with Housenka's care (see Chapter 6 for more details about Positive Health). In fact, Paul Klaassen, the first president of the Assisted Living Federation of America, and his partner Terry Klaassen—who co-developed the Assisted Living Home, the origin of Housenka, in the U.S., with Shigekazu Tanaka, Chairman of the Housenka Group—are also of Dutch ancestry. Our Assisted Living Homes are revolutionary nursing homes that combine aspects of U.S. nursing homes with Dutch group homes that provide housing and services to the elderly. The Netherlands also has some communities where entire towns are involved in dementia care, so there are many things we can learn from this model.

Innovative Dementia Care Methods Desired in This Age

The methods we have established will be described in detail in the next chapter and thereafter, but in brief, they consist of Logical Care (Fact Acceptance-Based Aid), Lateral Care (Reality Affirmation-Based Aid), and a fusion of the two, Integrative Care (Comprehensive Aid).

In developing these methods, we referred to previous studies and approaches to dementia care, such as validation, which builds a relationship of trust based on empathy with the person; Humanitude, which eases anxiety through words, eye contact, touch, and the like; and person-centered care, which considers the person's needs from their own perspective. However, the communication methods in which we observe the residents' words, behavior, and facial expressions, and at times, actively work to enter the resident's "reality" to understand them better and provide personalized and detailed care, are unique to Housenka.

The core goal of our methods is to provide on-site care that brings out the "will to live" in people with dementia and works to further improve their quality of life (QOL) so that they can lead their lives as smoothly as possible.

However, since dementia consists of complex and personalized symptoms, we cannot simply apply our care methods as a universal solution. The information in this book is just our principles and "functional equations" that are necessary to formulate appropriate care. Imputing a variety of variables into that function—such as the actual needs of the person with dementia, the person's cognitive symptoms and BPSD, personality, family situation, environment, and the presence of fluctuations—the output, which is the appropriate care for that individual, will show aspects unique to them and will be extremely different to care for others. We believe that this complexity and the variables involved is proof that the ultimate pursuit of functional care—which aims to draw out the power to live within each unique individual, by deriving personalized care through our care method function—is necessary for dementia care.

The attention that dementia receives in the future as a global issue will surely grow. As a country that is having to face the issues of a super-aging society earlier than others, we believe that Japan has the ability to establish new dementia care methods, and it is our purpose to spread these methods to the rest of the world.

Article #1

"Dementia Villages" Outside of Japan

One of our visions is to create a dementia care paradise in Japan. The development of similar concepts, such as operational communities where people live with dementia, have already started overseas.

Hogeweyk in the Netherlands and Village Landais Alzheimer in France are examples of such communities. In these communities, people with dementia can live and act as they wish without being restricted by social norms and conventions, and there are always people around to support them when they need help. I see these as the kind of ideal communities that we wish to create in Japan. Although it is not considered a dementia village, there is also a place called The Center for Discovery (TCFD), located about a two-hour drive from New York City. TCFD is a huge town-like complex that provides education, medical care, and housing for children with disabilities, as well as a wide range of support, from medical care and daily life to employment and housing, for adults who still require support. Fortunately, I was able to visit TCFD when I underwent a multi-day training program there. It is staffed by approximately 1,700 employees who support residents with a variety of physical, intellectual, and mental needs. Most of the staff are dressed like local residents and blend in with the environment. I remember liking the fact that the staff were not dressed like traditional nursing care supervisors or caregivers. The Center also includes a laboratory, where researchers from prominent U.S. universities gather to conduct various studies to make life as comfortable and peaceful as possible for the children and other residents who gather in this community. There were also farms, barns, movie theaters, supermarkets, and restaurants—most of which were built thanks to donations—within TCFD. These facilities were not only used by the disabled residents but were also staffed by them. In other words, the people at TCFD were living normal, everyday life. This is something that TCFD has in common with Hogeweyk and Village Landais Alzheimer, and another facility we can learn from when creating our vision of a dementia care paradise.

Hogeweyk and Village Landais Alzheimer has been criticized by some as being closed off or a fake paradise.

However, we believe that the purpose of dementia care is, in principle, to allow people with dementia to live independent and peaceful lives, where their words and actions are affirmed without restrictions or constrictions, their existence is respected, and they are free from stress and pain as much as possible. We also believe that this is the type of care that helps reduce the stress of caregivers. In our view, Hogeweyk and Village Landais Alzheimer are conducting a brilliant form of dementia care by providing a place where people with dementia can lead a peaceful life in a warm, welcoming, and reassuring environment.

Dementia villages were pioneered by the Netherlands and France, and now, they also exist in Norway, Denmark, Italy, and Australia. Plans are also underway in the United Kingdom and Canada.

Currently, nursing homes in Japan only consist of a single floor or a small part of a facility. Our hope is to create a dementia care paradise, where a whole community is devoted to care, as soon as possible.

Chapter 2
New Dementia Care

The "Downward Spiral" That Traps Families

Frustration From Answering the Same Questions Repeatedly

Let us take a look at a conversation that may take place between a grandfather with dementia and his family.

Shortly after the family eats lunch, the grandfather asks, "Did I eat lunch yet?"

"Yes. You just ate," answers a family member.

"Oh, alright," the grandfather says as he nods.

However, a few minutes later, he asks the same question.

"Did I eat lunch yet?"

Here we go again, thinks the family.

"You already ate. Although I already told you this earlier," the family points out in a light tone.

The grandfather answers as if he understands. After a few minutes, the grandfather repeats himself.

"Did I eat lunch yet?"

The third time causes the family's frustration to boil over.

"How many times do I have to tell you!? Enough is enough!"

This kind of conversation is common in many homes where a family member has dementia. Even in nursing homes, this is not an uncommon sight, although the tone of the conversation may be lighter. It is understandable to feel frustrated when someone asks you the same question repeatedly. However, in the case of someone with dementia, it makes no sense to get angry at them. As explained in the previous chapter, dementia is a functional disorder of the brain that causes memory loss.

Since memory problems are common symptoms of dementia, blaming the lack of ability, which is beyond their control, will not lead to an improvement in the situation. However, many caregivers confront the person with dementia in situations like this, which means that the caregiver does not understand the true nature of dementia. It may also mean that the caregiver understands but is too tired to respond appropriately.

To the grandfather, each time he asks the question, he believes it is the first time he is asking it. He has serious concerns about whether he ate lunch or not. When the answer to his question is "I told you earlier" or "enough is enough," the grandfather feels uncomfortable, uneasy, or even angry.

The stress of a negative response can cause the person with dementia to suffer, and it can lead to further exacerbation of their symptoms. Continuing care that does not lead to visible positive outcomes is difficult for any caregiver and adds to the burden of caregiving. As a result, the caregiver becomes even more stressed, and is more prone to responding negatively to the person with dementia, which further worsens the symptoms of dementia. There are actually many caregiving families that become trapped in this downward spiral.

When Support Becomes an Imposition

In general, there are two ways that families fall into this spiral.

The first is when the family has no knowledge about dementia. They do not understand why the person with dementia forgets so quickly and they try hard to make the person learn and remember things.

The other way is that the family is aware that dementia causes memory impairment, but the burden of caregiving causes them to forget this fact at times, and they end up responding inappropriately.

In fact, we have seen a good number of families who have tried to make a person with advanced dementia solve math drills, crossword puzzles, or the like. When the person with dementia was unable to solve the task, the family members scolded the person with dementia. It was a painful sight to see.

Another time, when we visited a home of a person with dementia, there were notes posted all over the house, such as "toilet is here," "snack in refrigerator," and "turn off the gas as follows." The family thought the person with dementia would be able to remember if everything was written down. Using visual clues, such as posting notes, is an effective way to support a person with dementia. In fact, as will be discussed in more detail in Chapter 3, there are cases where Housenka has used message cards to improve the lives of our residents.

However, in the case above, the person with dementia was no longer able to read, and in an environment full of unorganized information, instructions by family members would cause them to panic. Actions that cause confusion to the person does not count as support, and in harsher words, the caregiver is just forcing their wishes upon the person.

Chasing a Past Image

Since family members recall how the person with dementia was when healthy, it is understandable that they do not want to accept the current situation, and desire that the person return to how they were. The families who forced the person with dementia to solve drills and crossword puzzles did so out of a desperate desire to "cure" their loved ones. However, from an objective perspective, forcing a person to do something they cannot do only causes pain. There is no going back to the past, and fixating on the past images of your loved one does not help. It is important to understand the actual situation you are currently facing.

A negative reaction from family members is surely crushing for the person with dementia as well. If you care about the person with dementia, it is important not to chase the person's past image. dementia care begins with accepting the person with dementia as they are now. You must abandon your desire to make them remember, to teach them, or to cure them, because if you fall into a downward spiral like the example at the beginning of this chapter, the situation will worsen regardless of your intentions. The most important step of dementia care is to understand the characteristics of dementia, so you do not become trapped in a downward spiral.

Learning New Things Even With Dementia

While we have mentioned that it is not a good idea to try to make a person with dementia remember or teach them new things, there are cases when they are able to learn. Although it depends on the individual and/or circumstances, the ability to remember or memorize is not completely lost. Let's take a look at the following.

Housenka fully cooperated in a two-year demonstration project for an online travel service for care providers by NEC Solution Innovator Co., Ltd. (part of the Ministry of Economy, Trade, and Industry's "Effectiveness Verification Project of Products and Services for a Dementia-Inclusive Society") and conducted a trial of virtual reality (VR) travel for people with mild cognitive impairment (MCI) and mild dementia, lasting from September 2021 to March 2022 and from September 2022 to January 2023. For this demonstration project, users wore VR goggles to experience realistic simulations of an Awa Odori dance tour in Tokushima or a Miyajima tour in Hiroshima.

In the case of a man with MCI who participated in the project, he yelled at the staff angrily when we tried to have him wear the VR goggles, even though we explained everything thoroughly beforehand. However, as he enjoyed two or three VR trips, we noticed some changes. He was able to remember what the goggles were used for and started to willingly put the goggles on. When we discussed the VR trip three days after the last session, he could not remember the destination of the trip or conversations that took place. However, when we showed him the VR goggles, he was able to remember scenes from the trips such as riding a boat and trains in the background. He also participated in the project in the second year and is now enjoying VR trips very much. The staff on site has stated that due to the VR trips, he converses and interacts with others more, which in turn has led to less problems associated with memory.

An important factor is that the person with dementia enjoys the activity. While it is true that memory impairment gradually worsens in those with MCI or mild dementia, it does not mean that they cannot memorize or remember at all. From our experience, it seems that episodic memories, especially those acquired through experience, are relatively easier to retain. As stated earlier, the important thing is to not force anything. If caregiver actions cause the person with dementia to feel stressed, they are doing more harm than good. Caregivers must understand that due to the memory impairment, "the norm" or "common sense" may not apply to the person with dementia. Determining this fine border of their remaining abilities is an extremely important point in dementia care.

Pay Attention to Facial Expressions

We believe that the best outcome of dementia care is for "the person with dementia to lead an independent and peaceful life, free from stress and pain, according to their situation." Another, equally important point is reducing the stress of caregivers.

If care is not showing results despite best efforts, then make sure that the support is actually working. The facial expressions and behavior of the person with dementia is an important clue to determine whether or not the person is comfortable with the situation. The caregiver must pay attention to facial expressions and behaviors to gauge how effective their care is. If the person with dementia frowns, makes a gloomy face, ignores the caregiver, or tries to leave the area, it is likely that they do not understand what is being said, and the other person must try to convey their thoughts in a different way. On the other hand, if the person with dementia softens their expression or becomes calm, then the communication method is working. For communication between two healthy individuals, both parties can work to improve an issue, but this is often not possible for people with dementia. Therefore, it is necessary for the caregiver to decipher the person's thoughts and feelings through facial expressions and behavior and determine if the care being provided is appropriate or if there is a mismatch. This is the difference between "normal" communication and communication in dementia care.

Even Care Workers Become Trapped By Their Idea of "Ideal Care"

What Someone Cannot Do is More Noticeable Than What They Can Do

It is not only family members who tend to assume that if you teach or explain something to a person with dementia, they can easily do, remember, or understand it. In fact, many professional caregivers also fall into this trap. In particular, there are often cases in professional care settings where the caregiver focuses more on what a person cannot do, rather than what they are still able to do. For example, if a caregiver notices that the person cannot hold utensils properly when eating, the caregiver may take over and bring the food to the person's mouth; or the caregiver may hand a television remote to the person even if the person was able to do it themselves when given time.

We believe that the purpose of professional care is to support independence. Professional caregivers must determine what a person can do and guide them towards an independent life where they can use their remaining abilities as much as possible. Assistance and care should obviously be provided for tasks the person is unable to do or tasks that take too much time, but it is important to identify the person's ability and encourage them to use it in daily life. Such care is often difficult for family members to provide at home, and that is why the existence of professional caregivers are significant.

Going back to the person who is unable to hold utensils properly, the appropriate level of aid would be to hold the person's hand to support it as they bring the food to their mouth. If the person wishes to eat with their hands, caregivers can prepare a meal that can be eaten by hand so the person can eat on their own. In this case, the caregiver's job is to prepare hygienic meals with shapes and temperatures that considers the person's abilities. If a person is struggling to grab a remote, the caregiver can move it to a location on the table where the person can reach. This way, the person is still able to do part of the task.

People actually feel stressed if someone is doing everything for them all the time, and if that continues, they get tired of their daily routine.

When someone needs care, it means that others will be doing many things for the person whether they like it or not. That is why we believe that true care is about striking a balance between "having someone do something for the person" and "the person doing something for someone else." To make life as motivating as possible for the person, it is important to reduce the support given to them as much as possible while increasing tasks that the person can do for others.

Creating Situations Where Individuals Can Shine

However, looking at the actual situations in care, we feel that in addition to a lack of time and staff, there is a strong tendency to obsess about problems that could result from leaving things to the individual (i.e., injuries, accidents, schedule disruptions, etc.), and to immediately provide aid when a person is unable to do something.

It is understandable that watching a person with dementia slowly work on a task can be frustrating. However, eliminating the time for waiting and just watching the person leads to cold impersonal care. As a result, the person's ability is further undermined or weakened, and the person themselves will be in a "person-to-be-cared-for mindset," which reduces their motivation to live and makes them less independent. In short, the "care" provided is the opposite of actual lifestyle support.

As a professional caregiver, it is necessary to possess the ability to identify the person's motivation and abilities and provide care that draws them out. This may even lead the person to step into a position where they can help another person. It will lead to an increase in the person's self-confidence, self-efficacy, and sense of self-usefulness, which will greatly contribute to the improvement of QOL. For example, even if a person with dementia cannot perform a series of actions to complete a task such as making soup, by breaking down the process into smaller parts, you will notice that there are still many actions that the person with dementia can still do. In the case of making soup, this may be bringing the pot, cutting the ingredients, or pouring the soup into bowls. Even those who require assistance for daily tasks such as bathing and changing clothes may be able to help in other ways. A person who is still able to knit well can teach others how to knit, while a person good at singing can become a chorus leader.

Receiving gratitude or praise from others is an important factor for enjoying life. We believe that the challenge for professional caregivers is to determine each person's abilities and create opportunities where each individual can shine.

Three Habits of Thought that Create "Common Sense"

Unconsciously Acting Leads to Unbalanced Care

We have explained the "assumptions," "downward spirals," and the "idea of ideal care" that family members and professional caregivers tend to fall into, but the reason that people fall into these traps is common for all three. It is the mindset of trying to measure others according to our own senses, sensibilities, and values. In reality, the daily behavior of humans is based on mental models. A mental model is the subconscious mind of an individual that guides our thoughts, and includes assumptions, values, and common sense.

The mental model is formulated through an individual's past experiences, which form the basis for their thoughts, which in turn guides their words and actions. What is important to know is that there are three types of unintended mental movements that contribute to the formulation of a mental model: stereotyping, unconscious bias, and paternalism.

Stereotypes, or stylized common sense, are preconceptions based on assumptions and fixed views. Examples include "food must be eaten with utensils" or "people should only sleep on beds or futons." Humans make unconscious assumptions that enable us to make quick judgments and think fast. However, within this process is a distortion or bias in the way we see or perceive things that we are not aware of. This is what is referred to as unconscious bias.

Unconscious bias is an unwitting evaluation of a stereotype based on emotions and morals formulated through personal opinions and feelings.

Examples include "eating with your hands is embarrassing, dirty, and can lead to burns" or "sleeping on a sofa is not good for your health." In a long-term care setting, these views develop into ideas such as "if residents are doing such things, it will make it seem like we are not providing proper care." Caregivers who have such ideas may try to stop residents from eating with their hands at all costs or repeatedly attempt to have residents sleep in a bed.

Paternalism is when a professional or authority figure unilaterally supports a person (especially a vulnerable person) based on their own values without listening carefully to the person's wishes or story because they believe it is in the best interest of that person. An example would be doctors or caregivers trying to steer residents in a particular direction based on their own values. A caregiver who believes that serving three well-balanced and calorie-calculated meals a day is the key to health may continue to serve the same meals without considering the individual person's dietary patterns and preferences.

Mental Models May Be the Source of Stress for Caregivers

Humans acquire stereotypes, unconscious biases, and paternalism as natural or tacit knowledge in the course of our social life to create mental models. Since these become entrenched at the unconscious level, once acquired, it is difficult to change even when we encounter new events and experiences.

On the other hand, those with dementia are freed from the framework of such social norms and stereotypes and shift from living as part of society to living in a world of their own. For a person with dementia living as they wish, free from society's common sense and the norm, the mental models of caregivers are often a hindrance to the freedom of that person. Yet, oftentimes, caregivers stick to their values of common sense and what is ideal, and demand that the person act accordingly. The caregivers continue to believe ideas (such as "repeating things enough will help someone remember," "doing drills can help someone regain their ability to calculate," or "food must be eaten using utensils") and if the person with dementia acts contrary to these values, the caregiver may feel frustrated or respond negatively. This leads to a mismatch in care. When providing dementia care, it is necessary to recognize that the source of stress for caregivers lies in these "habits of thought" that are ingrained in the subconscious. This is true not only for families providing care at home, but all caregivers, including professionals working at nursing homes.

Recognizing Mental Models: A Paradigm Shift in Dementia Care

We believe that recognizing and becoming aware of the habits of thought mentioned in this chapter is the paradigm shift necessary in dementia care.

Unless we can free ourselves from stereotyped ideas and unconscious bias, the situation will not improve no matter how much we try to adapt to the individual circumstance of the person with dementia. If, for example, the person begins to eat with their hands, common sense will tell the caregiver to hand them a utensil, and if they are unable to use the utensil, assistance will be immediately provided. This is actually quite common in a general long-term care setting. Stereotyped ideas include:

"People must use utensils to eat."

"People must bathe."

"We must stop people from wandering."

"People must sleep in a bed at night."

These fixed thoughts of caregivers lead to unhappy dementia care for all because they cause frustration to the caregiver when these are not realized, which in turn increases the stress of the person with dementia and drives down quality of life. To clarify, this does not mean that the person with dementia should be left alone at all times, but rather that forcing them to fit a mold is not good for all parties involved.

If a caregiver can relax and tolerate behaviors that may not be the norm, it will lead them to be kinder to the person with dementia and more accepting of various feelings. This will result in calmer expressions by the person with dementia. If the person with dementia has been reluctant to take a bath, you can ask again when they are calmer. If they are calm in a certain situation, review the situation to make sure there are no dangers or risks and make the necessary environmental arrangements.

Being Aware of Our Perspectives

To bring our mental model, which is basically part of our unconsciousness, to the surface of our consciousness, it is important to be aware of our perspectives so we can view things in a different way, with a broader scope, and from a different position. By changing our perspective, a person with dementia will not only be "a person with a disease," but also "just like any other person" or "someone who is of use to others."

By broadening our perspective, we may be able to calmly explore why the individual is refusing care, or to step away for a moment to calm ourselves. Furthermore, by thinking about the situation in someone else's shoes, we can think about whether we are unknowingly putting our own convenience first in the line of daily work, or whether we are actually focusing on what the person with dementia needs and not just our own responsibilities.

The key is to change our way of thinking as such, to reach a unity of knowledge and action, where our awareness, actions, and practices are working in unison. We must always be aware that changing our way of thinking alone is difficult but implementing it will be even more difficult. To be honest, we at Housenka sometimes still tend to act according to our own mental models at times, even though we understand these concepts. However, knowledge of stereotypes, unconscious bias, and paternalism makes it easier to be objective about our mental behavior and to modify our behavior. In addition, we are constantly striving to move away from actions based on assumptions through training and mutual checking mechanisms. If people are not careful, they tend to view and judge the world through their own fixed perspectives. It is not easy to break free from this tendency, but we must overcome it to realize a paradise for those with dementia.

Common Problems in Care: Mismatch of Words and Actions

There is one more issue that caregivers must keep in mind. In the field of long-term care, there is a common way of doing various things, which many caregivers accept as a fixed model of some sort. This is especially true of professional caregivers. For example, in the morning, a caregiver enters a resident's room and says, "Good morning, did you sleep well?" and opens the curtains before the resident can reply. The caregiver continues to say, "I hear it's going to get hot today," but instead of choosing clothes according to the weather and the resident's mood, the caregiver simply presents the clothes that they set out the previous night. Another caregiver passes a resident in the hallway and nicely asks, "Have you eaten?" The resident replies "Yes," but before he can continue, the caregiver quickly leaves to do their next task.

What is common in the two examples above is that there is a discrepancy between the caregiver's words and actions. This type of discrepancy is actually quite common in the long-term care field. The reason why this happens is that a framework has been established for many aspects of long-term care, and the system is designed to provide care within the flow of daily routines. In this system, the flow of daily life follows a routine rather than changing according to the actions and reactions of the residents. Caregivers are taught to say "Good morning. Did you sleep well?" in the morning and open the curtains to encourage the residents to get up. Since the care they provide is following this model, the caregiver assumes that they are properly caring for residents.

Many times, caregivers are unable to notice that there is a mismatch between the knowledge of the caregiver and the actual care being provided. This phenomenon is a trap that is especially common among professional caregivers. Like the aforementioned habit of thought, this happens because the caregiver reaches a conclusion only through their own worldview, and it can lead to behavior that subconsciously disrespects the resident's existence.

When there is a discrepancy in a caregiver's words and actions, it can contribute to confusion and stress for the person with dementia. When this continues, it can lead to restlessness, verbal outbursts, loss of appetite, and the like. These reactions by the person with dementia cause the caregiver to become frustrated, and the frustration of not achieving desired outcomes despite their best efforts leads to stress and exhaustion for the caregiver.

There is nothing more pointless than a situation that does not reward either the person with dementia or the caregiver. To resolve this, it is essential to break the cycle of stress that is common in dementia care, and to do so, caregivers must not be influenced by common models of care. Caregivers must look at the facial expressions and actions of the individual with an unbiased eye and constantly review their own care to see if appropriate care is being provided. Such an attitude is essential in dementia care.

Past Dementia Care Is Wrong!

The Case of Mrs. Yamamoto: What We Realized As She Ate With Her Hands

As we can understand from the previous section, caregivers tend to apply their own "common sense" and "norm" when providing dementia care. Many professional caregivers in particular value the terms "user-oriented" or "customer-oriented," but in reality, they often act within their own mental model, and as a result, the care they provide is not actually user-oriented in many cases. In fact, we at Housenka used to make the same mistake, and were providing care based on our own "common sense" and "norm."

The person who made us realize our mistake was the 83-year-old Tamae Yamamoto (pseudonym), whom we mentioned in the "Introduction" section. According to her family, Mrs. Yamamoto was a dependable person when she was working as a nurse. Once she entered Housenka due to dementia, she often left her room at night to sleep on a sofa and was also frequently seen eating meals by hand. We saw these behaviors as detrimental for Mrs. Yamamoto and began to provide support under the assumption that helping her return to her former self would benefit her. For example, if she was sleeping on the sofa, we guided her back to her room so she could sleep on a bed, and if she was eating with her hands, we encouraged her to use utensils.

However, about a month after we started this support, we witnessed shocking sights that left us speechless. At Housenka's specialized nursing homes, cameras are installed in some common areas for security purposes, and with the consent of the families, cameras are installed in some of the residents' rooms for the research and development of dementia care. When we viewed the camera footage of Mrs. Yamamoto after she was led back to her room to sleep on her bed, she was just sitting on the edge of her bed in the dark with her head down. There was also footage of her stopping in place or her expression becoming stiff when forced to hold a utensil to eat. Furthermore, the staff started to report that she was refusing care, which had not been the case before, and that she was wandering at night more frequently. Her expressions and actions indicated that we were not providing the right kind of support.

This led us to thoroughly review our support. As a result, we realized that we had a fixed view about common sense in society and how people should act, and subconsciously rejected Mrs. Yamamoto's actions since they deviated from this view. This was the moment we became aware of our own internal stereotypes, unconscious bias, and paternalism. We were bound by our predetermined view and applied our ideas of "how a person should be" to Mrs. Yamamoto and evaluated her actions under this assumption.

As a result, we were actually totally denying her actions and behavior. It was very hard for us to admit this fact because it meant admitting that the care we worked hard and earnestly to provide was completely wrong. However, we had to face our mistakes to progress. We set out to improve every aspect of our support.

Our Revamped Care Brought Back Smiles to Mrs. Yamamoto's Face

According to her family, when Mrs. Yamamoto was a nurse, she used to take naps on a sofa during night shifts. We settled on the idea that if Mrs. Yamamoto has returned to that time of her life in her mind, sleeping in a bed is actually more unnatural for her. Therefore, we first accepted Mrs. Yamamoto's "reality." Our staff kept the sofa clean and sanitized, and when Mrs. Yamamoto fell asleep there, they covered her with a warm blanket and let her sleep there instead of leading her back to her room. We also decided that if she wanted to eat with her hands, we should not force her to use utensils. Instead, we cleaned her hands thoroughly and let the food cool down a bit before serving it to prevent her from burning her hands.

Once we changed our policy, Mrs. Yamamoto began sleeping soundly on the sofa and eating well. Above all, she began to look calmer and more animated, smiling and helping other residents by pushing their wheelchairs when they moved around. Although the care we provided to Mrs. Yamamoto is Functional Care that only applies to her, her case helped us realize many things, such as:

- the major discrepancy between our words and actions.

- how much we were restraining or denying our resident's actions.

- how our well-meaning care was actually depriving residents of their independence, freedom, and, more importantly, their smiles.

- how all of this was being conducted unconsciously without any bad intentions.

Long-term care based on the framework of common sense, if done incorrectly, can trample on the dignity and values of the person with dementia. This can lead to "correction" based on the caregiver's stereotypes which can further lead to "coercion." If we view a person with dementia as "inferior," we tend to fall under the illusion that "rescuing" that person from that state is a virtue. Rather, it is important to be aware that people with dementia have their own world and culture that differ from our common sense, and that in a sense, they are free of the social bonds that shackle us, and to recognize this as another form of diversity. We as caregivers must always pay attention to the support we provide and reflect on whether it is truly helping the person with dementia. We must be vigilant to ensure that we are not falling into bad habits of thought when caring for people with dementia. We believe that this is one of the most important professional skills for those who work in the field of human service, not only in the field of long-term care.

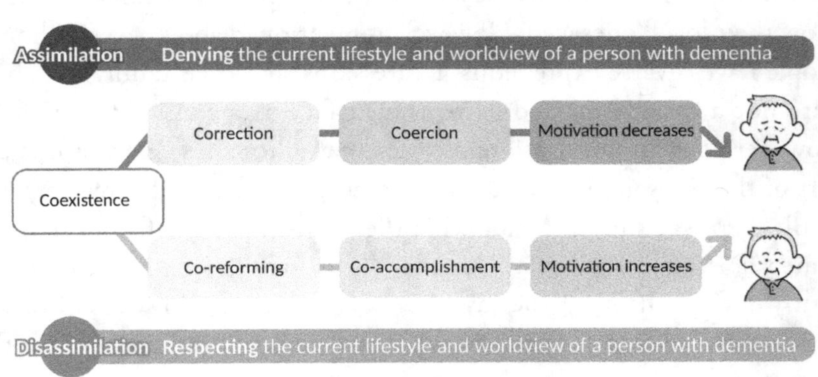

What Exactly is "Individuality"?

In the field of long-term care, it is often said that "it is important to respect the individuality of the person with dementia." I myself was taught this in the past, and I still want to respect the individuality of the person I am caring for. However, just like in Mrs. Yamamoto's case, as I gained more experience in the field, I came to realize that considering the person's "individuality" takes profound thought and is not something that we can talk about lightly. Even when I think about myself, I cannot immediately answer what I would consider my "individuality." I doubt there is anyone who can give an immediate answer.

Most people project different expressions according to the situation. The expression you project when you are with family, at work or school, or when alone is all different. Even when at home, your expression is different according to the situation, such as when enjoying time with family, scolding a child, or thinking about something. People with dementia also show a wide variety of expressions in different situations. They may be smiling when relaxing in the sunlight, or they may be angry and violent due to anxiety or fear. The expressions that caregivers see in the line of duty are only a small part of the person with dementia. I have come to believe that it is very dangerous to use one aspect of the individual to define what their "individuality" is, especially if it is based on the caregiver's subjective view.

Family members of people with dementia tend to assume that they know their loved ones well. However, as mentioned above, even at home, people have diverse expressions. Expressions that even family members were not aware of may come to the surface as a result of dementia. However, it is an unquestionable fact that all of these expressions are part of that person. To put it simply, neither professional caregivers nor family members should decide what the "individuality" of a person with dementia is. In a sense, "individuality" is like an illusion that cannot be clearly defined. If this is the case, I believe that the main focus of care is not to help the person return to their past state, but rather to accept the present and help the person live peacefully.

> "This is not my father's true self."
>
> "My mother didn't used to be like this."

These are some of the laments we hear from families of people with dementia. It is understandable that family members would respond like this. However, dementia care truly begins once families understand that organic changes in the brain due to dementia cause many changes and can accept those changes as part of their loved ones.

Focus on "As Is" Rather Than "Individuality"

This headline also applies to professional caregivers. Even professional caregivers become shackled by the past image of the person with dementia, which undermines the quality of dementia care. For example, assessment sheets are tools for reviewing lifestyle support for residents in elder care facilities. These sheets list the resident's name, address, basic information such as family structure, life history, medical history, employment history, house condition, and the like, as well as the current status of health conditions and physical and mental functions. Based on this information, caregivers think about the type of support that is desirable. In many cases, caregivers use these sheets as a guide to help the residents try to return to their previous state. However, it is important to refrain from providing this kind of support.

As previously explained, dementia is the result of irreversible changes in the brain. Therefore, it is impossible to restore a person with dementia to a past state no matter how hard caregivers try. While we believe it is meaningful to use these tools to understand the meaning of a person's words and actions, using it to try restoring that person's past "individuality" deviates from the essence of care. It is our opinion that rather than dwelling on the past, it would be more constructive and realistic to think about how to create a future plan for the person based on knowledge of the past. This is especially important since there are often cases where a person's preferences change due to dementia. For example, someone who used to like watching sumo wrestling will show no reaction even when a caregiver informs them that the sumo broadcast has started. Instead of focusing on the person's "individuality" (past preference for sumo), caregivers must accept the present "as is" (shows no interest in sumo) to plan for the future. We believe this is a necessary step in dementia care.

To reiterate, the desired outcome of our care is to "enable people with dementia to lead independent and peaceful lives without stress or pain as much as possible, while reducing the stress of caregivers." If caregivers are too focused on the vague concept of "individuality," they will not be able to provide constructive care, and caregivers will only become exhausted when their efforts prove to be futile. Caregivers must pay attention to the person's facial expressions and behavior at that moment, and make sure that the person is calm and comfortable at that moment. We believe that this is the foundation of dementia care, and that the accumulation of these small moments will lead to an improved quality of life. Accepting the person's current state is what leads to beneficial dementia care for all parties involved.

"I Was Trying Too Hard Back Then!"

Let us look at a case of a married couple restoring a healthy relationship after a change of mindset. The couple was in their 80s, and the husband had dementia. Initially, the wife, who was caring for her husband at home, actively tried to restore her husband's memory and kept reminding him about their past. She would point to herself and ask, "Don't you know who I am? How come you can't remember?" She kept trying to jog her husband's memory in many different ways. "You used to like this, right?" "We took a trip here. How can you forget?" "Do you know who this person is?"

However, none of these actions resonated with her husband. In fact, it only caused the husband to look depressed, and he started to talk less and less. These futile efforts caused the wife to become exhausted and filled with a sense of emptiness. She finally decided that she could no longer care for her husband at home, and the husband moved into Housenka. After seeing how we treated her husband, and after we told her several times that forcing him to remember, understand, or memorize is counterproductive because it makes him cower or become confused, she changed how she interacted with her husband. She would look for conversations she can have with her husband at that moment or agree with whatever her husband was talking about. Although these conversations had no continuity, and the husband would forget the details a few minutes later, he became softer and calmer.

Of course, there is no continuity of conversation, and what was said is forgotten a few minutes later, but the husband's attitude has become soft and calm as before, and now he continues to talk amicably with his wife who comes to visit him. These days, he would have friendly conversations with his wife whenever she visits.

The wife looks back on the time when she was taking care of her husband at home with a laugh, saying, "I was trying too hard back then." Although her husband's memory impairment has not improved, the couple was able to regain their tranquil time together once the wife was able to respect and accept her husband's current state. We believe that this is the greatest expression of love from this wife to her husband.

Change Mental Models Through Repeated Conscious Realizations

While some families are able to understand their own habits of thought and change their behavior, there are also many cases where professional caregivers are unable to break free from their idea of ideal care.

Since our assumptions and habits of thought are deeply ingrained in our mind, it is not uncommon for them to revert back to a previous state if left unchecked, even if we are able to make improvements. We have seen many cases where the caregiver has the proper knowledge regarding mental models but ends up imposing their ideal care when they are actually in the field.

We know this in our heads, but when it comes time to take care of people with dementia in the field, we often find ourselves trying to correct their behavior in the direction that we think they should behave. It is like staying up late even though you know you must get up early the next morning, and then feeling rushed the next morning. This may give you an idea about how difficult the unity of knowledge and action is.

To resolve this issue, we at Housenka have established several mechanisms. One of the ways we do this is by sharing case studies among the parties involved during on-site training and case study training and discussing ways to make improvements. In the process, we sometimes uncover biased thinking among our caregivers. The first step in breaking free from their own mental models is for everyone to share the realization that they are being dragged down by "common sense" and "the norm."

We also have a supervising training system. The professionals in the field (the supervisees) are guided by their supervisor, who is in turn guided by a senior supervisor, such as the facility director or general manager. By monitoring each of these professionals in a multilayered manner, it promotes different awareness at each level and deepens the quality of guidance.

If you are taking care of a loved one at home, it is a good idea to share information about successful and unsuccessful care among family members, and to check with each other to see if anyone is bound by "common sense" or "the norm." Of course, consulting experts like us is also an option.

From our experience, age or experience does not factor into how quickly one can become aware of their own mental model. It is not necessarily true that veteran caregivers are able to recognize their habits of thought and put new models into practice more quickly than newcomers, and some newcomers are able to quickly act without being shackled by their own habits of thought. These individual differences are what makes care difficult.

Truly Preserving the Dignity of Those With Dementia

If caregivers are not careful, they tend to seek outcomes based on their own habits of thought. However, we believe that caregivers must overcome this to provide ideal dementia care. We define ideal dementia care as a setting where everyone's existence is positively accepted, and their will to live is supported until the end of their lives.

We explained earlier that professional caregivers must focus on what the person can still do, and draw out their abilities as much as possible, but this is also another example of something that is easier said than done.

People with dementia may not be able to express their needs and opinions well through words or actions. However, they still have emotions, ideas, and opinions. For example, even behaviors that seem inappropriate—such as removing their diapers at inappropriate times, eating with their hands, or taking someone else's food—are based on that person's own ideas and thoughts. However, such behaviors are considered "troublesome" by the caregivers, and they may be warned or stopped. In a general sense, those behaviors are inappropriate so it would be natural to stop them. But for the person with dementia, there is a reason for behaving that way, so they will not be able to comprehend why they are being told to stop.

No one enjoys it when their behavior is repudiated. This is also true for people with dementia. Just like anybody else, they want people to understand that their actions have meaning and purpose and want their current condition to be acknowledged and accepted. Caregivers must strive to understand the meaning and purpose of all behaviors of the person with dementia, affirm the person and support their will to live until the end. We believe that this is what "truly preserving dignity" means.

We are well aware that the long-term care field is short-staffed, time-pressed, and prone to stressful situations where things do not go as planned. But we must never forget that the desired outcome of care is to support the independence of people so they can lead a happier life. Even if things do not turn out as scheduled, it is not a major issue. The care will not mean anything if we neglect our main goal just so we can adhere to the schedule. By always being aware that this goal is the root of our care, our work will be rewarding, which helps reduce stress.

The person with dementia should use their remaining abilities as much as possible. Our job as caregivers is to aid them as necessary while searching for further remaining abilities. This type of lifestyle can help that person regain self-confidence and allow them to use their abilities to help others. The sense of self-efficacy and self-love gained leads to happiness for the person with dementia.

As mentioned earlier, an important step in discovering a person's remaining abilities is to break down actions and behaviors into smaller steps. For example, the task of "cleaning," consists of actions such as "putting away objects," "dusting," "vacuuming," and "mopping." If we think of all these actions as one, then that person may not be able to "clean," but she may be able to do the smaller actions such as dusting and mopping.

As in this example, there is usually something that the person can still do. Caregivers must broaden their perspective when assessing the person's remaining abilities. Assuming that all abilities were lost will not do any good.

The Three New Methods
That Will Change the Definition of Care

The Three Methods That Will Bring a Major Shift to Dementia Care

As we mentioned earlier, caring for Tamae Yamamoto (pseudonym) gave us insights that overturned many values we had previously believed to be correct, and. After 16 years of research and practice, we established two new methods for dementia care, and over the next two years, we developed a third method that combined the first two methods. These three methods are what we believe will bring a paradigm shift to dementia care. The three methods are: Logical Care (Fact Acceptance-Based Aid), Lateral Care (Reality Affirmation-Based Aid), and Integrative Care (Comprehensive Aid). The following is an outline of the three methods. We will explain in more detail in later chapters.

Logical Care (Fact Acceptance-Based Aid)

This method is aimed towards residents who are confused because they are unclear about the current situation they are in (objective facts) due to dementia. The caregivers repeatedly inform the residents of objective facts in a manner that they can understand so the resident can accept "facts" and understand their current situation.

To understand this concept better, try imagining yourself in that position. Events flow chronologically from the past to the present and from the present to the future. Since we understand the flow of events, we are able to comprehend and accept the current situation to decide our next action. However, we too may struggle to understand and accept the situation if something unexpected happens. In the case of people with dementia, their memories are not only vague but also full of gaps. Therefore, situations that may seem natural to us—since we understand the full chronology of the events—will confuse people with dementia because to them, a situation suddenly appears before them. In addition, to help people with dementia understand the facts that are before them, caregivers must organize the situation and information, and communicate it to them in a way they can understand, considering that dementia impairs comprehension and reasoning skills. The goal of Logical Care is to help the person with dementia to comprehend and accept the facts in front of them while taking the above into consideration.

Lateral Care (Reality Affirmation-Based Aid)

This method is aimed towards residents who are unable to comprehend objective facts. The caregivers work to understand what is in the mind of the person with dementia and provide support according to each situation. However, the scenes in their head and their thoughts do not necessarily flow in a straight line and can jump all over the place, so caregivers must channel into the current "reality" of the person with dementia when providing support.

Again, try imagining yourself in that situation. The caregiver uses Logical Care to explain the current situation to you in a simple manner, but to you, it seems as if no one is trying to understand the situation you are seeing and keeps disagreeing with your words. A healthy person may notice something wrong and assess the situation. But since memory does not flow chronologically for a person with dementia, they are unable to notice that something is wrong. To them, the people around are talking about another dimension, which causes the person with dementia to become confused by a variety of negative emotions such as anxiety, frustration, sadness, and anger. The goal of Lateral Care is to understand and accept that the person views the world differently, step into their "reality" to comfort them in order to help them comprehend the situation.

Integrative Care (Comprehensive Aid)

This method integrates the best parts of Logical Care and Lateral Care to provide support. For some people with dementia, either Logical Care or Lateral Care may be beneficial depending on the situation, scene, and time. For those types of residents, we observe their reactions to the situation and provide the right type of care accordingly.

Changing Care Depending on the Reaction

For those who are able to accept the "facts" if explained to them, we promote understanding through Logical Care by helping them comprehend the chronologically broken objective facts to reduce confusion and live as comfortably as possible. However, for those who are more confused if "facts" are explained to them, Lateral Care is used to detect the person's "reality" so that the caregiver channels into that "reality" and helps the person live comfortably within that "reality."

As a general rule, first we provide Logical Care to observe the person's level of understanding and acceptance of "facts." What is important to remember during this step is that the person does not need to fully understand the objective facts or continue to remember them indefinitely. The only criterion is whether or not the person can comprehend objective facts at the time. If the person is unable to accept the "facts" or shows confusion, we revise our communication methods, and if the person is still unable to accept the facts, we switch to Lateral Care.

In addition, as mentioned above, some people require different methods of care depending on the occasion or situation. For those people, we provide care from multiple angles through Integrative Care rather than strictly applying one method of care.

By applying different methods depending on the person, our aim is to realize an environment that is as stress-free as possible and support their will to live until the end. This is the new form of dementia care that we wish to achieve. The goal is not to forcefully apply one of these methods, but to help the person with dementia live comfortably. If our care does not seem to be working, we will change the method of care by observing the person's reactions, such as facial expressions, words, and actions, rather than trying to make the person adapt to our methods. We may have to use different methods for different people, different situations, and even with each passing moment. The resourcefulness and flexibility of care is the actual key to these methods.

Determine the Appropriate Method for the Person Through Assessment

A thorough assessment is necessary to identify the right method for the person and the situation. As already explained, the behavioral and psychological symptoms of dementia (BPSD) are complex and differ by person. Therefore, careful assessment is essential to determine the application of the three methods. At Housenka, we spent over a year developing an original assessment sheet, which we use to conduct our assessments.

Our assessments determine the person's level of understanding, including comprehension of explanations, visual and auditory comprehension, and mirror self-recognition, in addition to past medical history, time of onset of dementia, and physical and cognitive issues that are present. We determine which method of care to provide depending on the results of this assessment. However, this determination is extremely difficult. For example, we at Housenka have developed a "Seven-Stage Alzheimer's Disease Progression Chart for Residents of Housenka," but we cannot simply decide that Logical Care should be applied for residents up to a certain stage and Lateral Care should be applied for anyone above that. We determine the method that is appropriate for the person based on careful assessment and the past knowledge and experience of our caregivers and adjust based on the resident's response. As we continue to provide care, we can determine situations when Logical Care or Lateral Care was effective and apply them thereafter in similar situations.

In the case of Lateral Care, there is a need to know the person's life history as much as possible so caregivers can tune into the person's "reality." To this end, we interview the person and their family members to learn information such as where the person was born and raised, their job history, hobbies, and preferences. This information is recorded on the assessment sheet. In addition, we work to collect other subtle information for the assessment sheet, such as common behaviors, remarks, and facial expressions, locations in the facility where they are often seen, people who often appear in their conversations, people they are compatible or incompatible with in the facility, and monikers they respond to.

Naturally, the assessment is not done only once but is repeated on an ongoing basis, depending on the progress of symptoms, changes in relationships within the facility, and the like. If a resident who was receiving Logical Care now has difficulty understanding, or they stopped listening to or accepting explanations, it is not appropriate to continue forcefully providing Logical Care. It is important for the caregivers to always pay attention to the residents' facial expressions, speech, and behavior, and to have a keen eye to determine whether the support they are providing is appropriate.

TABLE 1: *Housenka's Seven-Stage Alzheimer's Disease Progression Chart for Residents*

Stage	Major Symptoms
Stage 1 No cognitive impairment (functions normal)	• Changes in the brain have begun, but there is no change in cognitive ability and no interference with daily living • Problems were not found during interviews with medical professionals, and the person and the people around believe the situation to be perfectly normal
Stage 2 Very mild cognitive decline (normal changes associated with aging or the first signs of Alzheimer's disease)	• Some lapse of memory • Cannot recall familiar words or names of family members or relatives • Forgets the location of items used on a daily basis such as keys and eyeglasses • Usage of pronouns such as "that" and "this" increases in conversations • Partially forgets the conversation after hanging up the phone • After making a schedule to meet up with someone, the person remembers the appointment itself, but cannot remember the date, time, or place • Forgets the destination or minor accidents increase while driving • Lose track of the story of a drama series or movies • The person or family members start to complain of memory loss
Stage 3 Mild cognitive decline (early stage of Alzheimer's disease)	• Loses track of days of the week, dates, and times • Cannot remember the names of new people • Repeats the same conversation from a few minutes ago or asking the asks the same question over and over

Stage	Major Symptoms
Stage 3 (cont'd)	<ul><li>Can hardly remember the contexts of texts</li><li>Loses or misplaces important items such as bankbooks, wallets, and personal seals</li><li>Ability to plan and organize decreases</li><li>Emotional expression and motivation decreases</li><li>Loses interest in hobbies and learning, and is often apathetic all day long</li><li>Makes more mistakes in the workplace and cannot perform duties as well as before</li><li>Becomes lost, runs red lights, and rear-end collisions increase while driving</li><li>Forgets how to use a TV remote</li><li>Friends, family members, co-workers, and others start to notice that something is obviously wrong</li></ul>
Stage 4 Moderate cognitive decline (diagnosed as mild or early stages of Alzheimer's disease)	<ul><li>Unable to manage money (settlements, payments, etc.)</li><li>Unable to perform somewhat difficult mental calculations (e.g., continuing to subtract 7 starting from 100)</li><li>Forgets memories of one's upbringing</li><li>Forgets or has a hard time remembering the current month or season</li><li>No longer able to tell what a TV remote is (semantic amnesia)</li><li>Has difficulty thinking of recipes, cooking, and choosing a menu item</li><li>Becomes uncomfortable in social situations and mentally challenging situations or becomes withdrawn</li></ul>
Stage 5 Somewhat severe cognitive decline (diagnosed as moderate or intermediate stage Alzheimer's disease)	<ul><li>Cannot recall important information such as home address, phone number, or their alma mater</li><li>Becomes confused about current location, date, time, day of the week, season, etc.</li><li>Unable to perform relatively simple mental calculations (e.g., continuing to subtract 2 starting from 40, continuing to subtract 2 starting from 20)</li><li>Cannot choose appropriate clothing for the season, situation, etc.</li><li>Can remember names of important people such as themselves, their spouse, and their children</li><li>Usually does not require assistance in eating or using the toilet</li><li>May need some convincing to bathe</li></ul>

Stage	Major Symptoms
Stage 6 Severe cognitive decline (somewhat severe or intermediate stage Alzheimer's disease)	• Almost completely unable to recognize recent experiences, events, and surrounding environments • Cannot completely remember their own upbringing, but can usually remember their own name • Sometimes goes outside alone, wanders, and gets lost • May forget names of important people such as their spouse, but can still tell apart the faces of acquaintances and strangers • Requires assistance dressing properly and may wear shoes on the wrong side • Failure to clean up after themselves after using the toilet, such as forgetting to flush or wipe • Excretes in places other than the toilet, increased frequency of urinary or fecal incontinence, requiring assistance to use the toilet • Refuses to bathe or needs assistance to bathe • Significant changes in personality and behavioral symptoms such as suspicions, delusions, hallucinations, and obsessive or repetitive behaviors
Stage 7 Very severe cognitive decline (severe or late-stage Alzheimer's disease)	• Unable to recognize the face of spouses and children • Becomes unresponsive when spoken to or facial expressions become stiff • Eyes are often closed and stops smiling • Can only understand or speak a few simple words such as "yes" • Loses control of physical functions and becomes bedridden, and symptoms such as dysphagia, muscle stiffness, and abnormal reflex reactions appear

Note: Based on a system developed by Barry Reisberg, M.D., New York University School of Medicine; supervised by Kazuhide Nishiyama, M.D and Manabu Fukuhara, M.D of Housenka Clinic.

Removing Stress for the Person With Dementia is Important

The main goal of using these three methods, and the challenge for us in our quest to create a dementia care paradise, is to remove stress for the people with dementia. Stress is an obstacle to a healthy and motivated life for all people, but healthy people can relieve their stress or work to remove what is causing stress. People with dementia experience anxiety about their fading memories, frustration at not being able to communicate their intentions and thoughts, and difficulty in understanding and processing situations appropriately, which itself causes stress. They also feel high stress just from daily living. And unfortunately, their declining abilities make it difficult to relieve the stress on their own. Therefore, we added a section on the assessment sheet entitled "Identification of Stressors." In this section, we check and quantify our residents' stress levels in six categories: natural environmental stress (weather, climate, etc.), social stress (relationships, etc.), mental stress (anxiety, anger, etc.), physical stress (illness, lack of sleep, etc.), facility-related stress (room, lighting, noise, etc.), and other stress (meals, pollen, etc.). Using this data, we create a stress radar chart and analyze in detail the areas where the residents are feeling the most stress.

Based on this overall information, we make a comprehensive assessment of the obstacles in the residents' life, and whether or not it is reducing their quality of life. For example, suppose a resident often wanders around the facility during the day. If they seem calm while wandering, we will allow the wandering to take place since it is not reducing their quality of life. However, if the wandering causes problems with other residents, it will lead to a decline in quality of life, so we would conduct measures to eliminate the risk.

After implementing these care plans that we drafted, we evaluate whether or not the support was effective, and conduct a reassessment. This includes a review of the resident's independence and cognitive function, an interview of the resident and family members, and a check of the resident's "facial expressions." This check of the resident's "facial expression" is the point we focus on the most. We evaluate whether we are truly achieving the support that the resident desires by comparing photos of the resident to see how their facial expressions have changed from the beginning of the stay to three months later. This comparison is conducted periodically.

Since introducing the three methods along with the detailed assessment, we have noticed that the facial expressions of our residents have gradually become calmer, more cheerful, or more peaceful.

Dementia Care Must Merge Knowledge and Creativity

Caregivers must acquire basic dementia knowledge, understand the individual situation of the person with dementia, and change their response according to the person's reactions. We believe that the outcomes of dementia care will only be evident after this process is repeated many times. The key is how the caregivers provide support. We hope that readers will use the information about Logical Care, Lateral Care, and Integrative Care that is introduced in the next chapter as specific hints when providing care.

As mentioned earlier, the basic premise for these methods is to understand that people are bound by mental models and have the awareness to break free from them. Otherwise, it will not be possible to truly provide care that respects the individual. What we want caregivers—whether they are family members or professionals—to realize is that dementia care requires a combination of knowledge and creativity. Care based only on knowledge will be excessively theoretical while care based only on creativity will be egocentric. Knowledge in this sense refers to "science," while creativity can be defined as "art." We will discuss the relationship between science and art in more detail in Chapter 6, but first make sure that you understand that the essence of dementia care lies in creative ideas that are produced on the spot.

Article #2
Autism Spectrum Disorder Care and the Effectiveness of "Structured Teaching"

Although it may seem surprising, dementia and autism spectrum disorder (ASD) care share some commonalities. Both of these conditions have many causes and encompass a wide range of symptoms, so the situation differs by the individual. Although the main symptoms are different, they are similar in that confusion caused by difficulties in communication can interfere with daily life and social interaction.

In short, care for dementia or ASD both require an understanding of the characteristics of the condition, and establishing communication and improving the living environment are the essential factors to improve quality of life. Therefore, it is no surprise that methods for ASD care can also be useful for dementia care. Since both conditions can be defined as cognitive functional impairments, there are inevitably many similarities in the methods of care.

In particular, we believe that "structured teaching," one aspect of the University of North Carolina TEACCH Autism Program, is also very effective in supporting people with dementia. For common cognitive impairments such as inability to understand the current situation well, inability to predict the future, peculiar obsessions, or worldviews, or being unbound by social norms, a structured visual approach has been evaluated as useful not only in supporting individuals with ASD, but also in supporting the lives of those with dementia. Specifically, this includes (1) physical structuring, which involves designating areas for specific tasks and creating a calm environment; (2) schedule structuring, which visually clarifies the schedule and clearly shows where events will take place; (3) communication structuring, which uses text, diagrams and illustrations; and (4) work system structuring, which visualizes work procedures such as the objective and method, and when the task is considered complete in order to help people perform better in life.

These are effective not only for people with ASD, but also for people with dementia who receive Logical Care and even those who receive Lateral Care.

To put it simply, structuring is the process of organizing information in a concise manner and devising ways to convey that enable those with communication impairments to understand and improve the living environment.

For example, if you enter a restaurant while on vacation to a foreign country and the menu is only available in the native language, you will not be able to tell what kind of food is offered. However, if the menu has pictures of the dishes, you will be able to have a clearer image of what is offered. This can be considered a form of "structuring." Structuring is also used in various other situations in daily life as a means to help people understand concepts without words, such as color-coded subway lines or the lines for bank ATMs.

Chapter 3
Practical Tips for Logical Care

The Key is to Support "Understanding"

Provide Support so the Person Can Accept Facts

In this chapter, we will explain Logical Care (Fact Acceptance-Based Aid) in detail and introduce cases where Logical Care was applied. Logical Care is a method where caregivers provide objective facts to a person who is confused due to dementia and then support the person so that they can accept the facts.

In general, "facts" refer to objective matters that have actually occurred and remain unchanged regardless of perspective. However, when a person's comprehension, memory, judgment, and ability to think abstractly deteriorate due to dementia, they may not be able to accurately accept facts, which will lead to confusion in their daily lives. Under the Logical Care method, we convey the "facts" to confused residents and help them accept the "facts" and regain a sense of satisfaction in their daily lives.

"Logical" means "according to logic or based on reason," and the term "logical thinking" refers to a form of vertical thinking, or the method of deepening ideas through sequential logical assessments. As such, our Logical Care method is one based on logic, where the support provided is logically connected chronologically, sequentially, or the like by a single line (context).

Although many people may be oblivious of the fact, we humans in fact have the ability to understand the current situation in the context of the flow of time: past, present, and future. In other words, we know that the current situation is connected to past events and have a broad idea of what it may lead to in the future because we can think of events in chronological or sequential order. This allows us to accept the current situation—or facts—without confusion.

However, dementia sometimes distorts a person's perspective of the flow of time, which makes it difficult to understand the "facts" that are currently occurring in front of them.

Logical Care supports the vertical thinking of such individuals and helps them to accept the current facts. If the person is confused because they cannot understand the facts, the caregiver will convey the facts in various ways each time to increase understanding and acceptance.

Some people may continue to understand or accept facts after they have done so once, while others may only be able to do so for a short time. It is fine if the understanding or acceptance only lasts momentarily. Logical Care is not intended to teach and make people remember, so please do not seek excessive outcomes based on such wrong assumptions. Its true purpose is to promote understanding and acceptance for the current situation, so that the person with dementia can smoothly transition to their next action. This is something all humans do subconsciously; we ourselves cannot move on to the next action without understanding and accepting the current situation.

In Principle, Start With Logical Care

Let's say there is a resident who is worried about whether they have already eaten or not. By telling the resident that they have just eaten, the caregivers encourage the residents to accept the fact that they have already eaten. The support can be considered as effective if the resident accepts the facts fully or at least partially.

Helping a resident who is in a nursing home but does not understand that fact and who expresses a desire to go home, by telling them the fact that the facility is now their home in a way that they can accept is also a form of Logical Care. In some cases, a resident's readiness to accept facts fluctuates throughout the day. For example, they may be able to accept facts easily in the daytime but not at night.

Caregivers must determine whether a resident is accepting facts through their responses. For example, let's say the caregiver tells the resident the current date. If the resident is able to accept facts, they will acknowledge that fact and respond normally. When the caregiver continues the conversation by saying, "It's the fifth year of the Reiwa (the current era of Japan; 2019–)," the resident may respond by saying, "Wow, it's already been five years since Reiwa started!" However, if the resident is unable to accept facts, when the caregiver says, "It's the fifth year of the Reiwa," the resident may respond by saying, "What's a Reiwa!?" If this happens, the caregiver should try to gather more information by asking the resident whether they know about Heisei (the previous era of Japan; 1989–2019). If they seem confused and think that the current era is Showa (1926–1989), it means that it is a different era according to the resident's "reality." In such cases, we will switch to Lateral Care (Reality Affirmation-Based Aid), in which we affirm the resident's "reality" and provide care while stepping into and becoming a part of their "reality."

When providing dementia care, in principle, we start with Logical Care to check the resident's communication abilities. If this does not work, or if Logical Care does not apply to the situation and it confuses the resident, we switch to Lateral Care or Integrative Care (Comprehensive Aid).

The appropriate method will vary depending on the individual and the situation, but in all cases, the goal is for the person with dementia to feel affirmed, secure, and safe.

Beware of Hearing Impairments: Convey Information Visually

The goal of Logical Care is to help residents understand facts through communication, but there are some key points to keep in mind when implementing it.

One is to focus more on communicating through vision rather than hearing. Many elderly people have some degree of hearing impairment. This means that in some cases, they are unable to hear or mishear the caregiver's words, leading to incoherent conversations. This may result in a person being diagnosed as lacking comprehension or judgment. Not being able to hear and not being able to understand are two very different things. We feel as if sometimes there are cases where those with hearing impairments who were misdiagnosed can develop actual dementia if the impairment is left untreated.

The following is a true story about a resident of Housenka. A short time after the resident entered Housenka, they were taken to an otolaryngologist who found earwax so large that it was blocking his ear canals. Once the earwax was removed, the resident was able to have conversations normally. It turned out that the resident's hearing impairment was simply a result of the earwax, and that their dementia was not actually that advanced. Cases such as this are not uncommon, so we recommend providing ear cleaning for any elderly person with suspected dementia—especially those who will be receiving Logical Care—before diagnosis.

However, there are still a certain number of people who have poor hearing even if their ears are cleaned. Some may be using hearing aids that do not fit them. Some people can hear normally but may often mishear words. Therefore, unless a person's hearing is very clear, it is recommended to provide information not only through hearing but also through sight. Examples include communicating through writing, putting up signs, and marking important daily life locations (e.g., toilet, location of clothes, etc.).

Another key point when implementing Logical Care is to communicate in a simple manner. Complicated statements such as, "First do this, then do that, and finally do this" are a source of confusion. Instructions for the person and facts they need to understand should be conveyed in a straightforward, focused manner. If possible, use simple phrases that alert the person and/or pictograms (simplified pictures or symbols that show information) rather than full complete sentences to increase understanding and comprehension.

Encourage Independence by "Structuring" the Living Environment

In Chapter 2, we introduced a case where the family of a person with dementia posted many notes throughout the house, which only caused the person to panic. While posting notes is good in terms of visual communication, there is room for improvement in this case if we take into consideration the basic principle of keeping information as simple as possible. At the same time as determining the key points of the person's daily life routines, it is also necessary to organize the living environment by removing unnecessary objects.

A contrasting care method would be one where the person's belongings are completely taken away, or the person is kept in an empty space (confined) during daytime hours. In fact, some medical and elder care facilities actually provide care in such bleak environments based on the idea that residents will be safe and will not panic if nothing is around them. However, such strange environments will also be a source of confusion for the residents, and above all, are not environments where people can stay comfortably.

At Housenka, residents can bring their own belongings and familiar furniture into their rooms. For those who are unable to organize their belongings by themselves, we will organize it for them. It is important to remove unnecessary objects, keep interesting but nonessential objects out of sight, and put away dangerous items such as magnets and thumbtacks, as well as detergent, soap, and other items that should not be eaten, to maintain a living space that is as comfortable as possible.

In some cases, those who are unable to organize themselves have been able to complete simple tasks such as putting their dirty clothes in the laundry basket, through the successful use of posted notes. This is a technique called "structuring," which we introduced in the article Autism Spectrum Disorder Care and the Effectiveness of "Structured Teaching" (Chapter 2). As mentioned in the article, it is often used to support autistic people to make their lives easier, but we believe it is also effective for dementia care and have incorporated it into our methods.

Humans constantly organize the information they receive from their surroundings, to understand the current situation and make a wide variety of decisions. However, people with dementia or autism have difficulty organizing and digesting the information from their surroundings. They are unable to determine why they are in the current situation or predict future events, so they tend to become anxious and panic. Devising ways to present information physically, visually, and temporally, can help people with dementia or autism to understand facts and live independently. For example, partitions can be used to reduce unnecessary information and stimuli and make it easier to understand the purpose of each space, or illustrations can be used instead of verbal instructions to convey the message in a clearer way.

Logical Care Case Studies

The following are actual examples of Logical Care in practice.

Case 1 Fixing the Failures of Initial Measures: Careful Explanation Leads to Acceptance of Facts

Eiko Ueyama (pseudonym), age 82, had Alzheimer's disease and lived alone. Her family noticed that her short-term memory and judgment was deteriorating through behaviors such as buying the same items multiple times, forgetting how to use detergent, losing the ability to manage her medications, and contacting her children multiple times a day for the same reason. The daughter decided that moving her mother to Housenka was the best option. Mrs. Ueyama's dementia was at Stage 4 according to Housenka's dementia progression chart. However, during the pre-move-in interview, Mrs. Ueyama would say that she can take care of herself and was confident that she can continue to live alone. She was completely unaware that she had dementia.

This made the daughter worry that her mother would stubbornly refuse if advised to move to a nursing home, and lead to broken relationships within the family. The daughter concluded that her mother needed to be tricked to enter the facility. Her plan was to repeatedly invite her mother to the restaurant in Housenka by telling her that it was a restaurant in a "hotel," eat there and return home. On the day of the actual move-in, they would eat at the restaurant like always, but instead of returning home, the daughter would tell Mrs. Ueyama that they will be staying at the "hotel" for the night. While our caregivers led Mrs. Ueyama to her room, the daughter would secretly go home to complete the move-in without Mrs. Ueyama noticing.

When we heard this plan from the daughter, we intuitively had a bad feeling. We tried to convince the daughter that her mother would be able to accept the move if she was told the truth directly. However, the daughter was concerned that if her mother—who is no longer able to live alone—refused to move in, there would be changes to her own life as well. She rejected our proposal and decided to carry out her own plan.

As the daughter had planned, on the move-in date, she was able to lead her mother smoothly to the residential floor after finishing their meal. The daughter then told her mother that they would be staying here today, and quietly left the area. Mrs. Ueyama was led into her room by our caregivers, but she got suspicious when she saw her own belongings—which should be at home—inside the room. Even though the caregivers tried to convince her that she was only staying for a night, she would anxiously and confusingly ask, "Why am I staying here?" "Where did my daughter go?" "Why is my furniture here?" and the like.

We felt that this situation would only increase the stress on Mrs. Ueyama, so we suggested to her daughter that we switch to Logical Care and tell Mrs. Ueyama the truth. The daughter hesitated, fearing that Mrs. Ueyama would become even more distraught, but in the end, she agreed. The caregivers politely explained the situation by saying, "You are actually having trouble living alone at home, and your family is worried about you. So, arrangements were made for you to move here to Housenka, where elders can live in peace." Mrs. Ueyama seemed to still have some doubts and anxiety, but she accepted the facts and calmed down.

When Mrs. Ueyama first moved in, she would ask, "Why am I here?" every few minutes but she would be satisfied each time when the reason was clearly explained. As time went by, the frequency of asking this question would decrease to once every few hours. Although she still occasionally asks, she has become accustomed to life at Housenka and now enjoys socializing with the other residents.

In this case, the initial measures failed because the family and we, the caregivers, assumed that Mrs. Ueyama would not be able to understand or accept the facts, without properly assessing her ability to understand. This case reminded us of the importance of first providing Logical Care to help residents accept the facts and then changing to Lateral Care only if that resident has difficulty comprehending the facts. Mrs. Ueyama's family told us that, "I thought it would be difficult for her to leave her home and live at the facility, but I was surprised at how easily she accepted it when the facts were conveyed to her truthfully. Seeing her getting along with other residents makes it feel as if my mother's sociable personality has returned, even though her cognitive symptoms have progressed."

While we initially went along with the daughter's strong desire to trick her mother in this case, a poor attempt at deception will only increase the discomfort for those who are still aware of the current situation to a certain extent, so explaining the facts truthfully may be the best action to take. However, it is important to explain the situation in a way that is easy to understand.

We completely understand a family's desire not to confuse the person with dementia. In fact, there have been cases in which family members have told a person truthfully about entering a facility, only to have the person firmly refuse to enter. As we have said many times before, there is no universal solution. What is important is to think about ways to convey information in a way that the person accepts, and the type of care desirable after moving in so that the person can adjust to the facility as soon as possible.

To carefully assess the best way to compromise, it is a good idea to include elder care experts such as the facility staff when discussing the arrangements for moving in, rather than just discussing it amongst one's own family.

Case 2 Patiently Conveying Facts: Improvement in Delusions of Theft

Masako Shimada (pseudonym), age 89, had delusions of theft even before entering Housenka. Although Mrs. Shimada's bankbook and other valuables were kept by her niece, Mrs. Shimada would often hysterically claim her bankbook was stolen and try to contact the police even after entering Housenka. We determined that telling Mrs. Shimada—whose memory and comprehension were impaired—the facts would be too confusing, so we decided to provide Lateral Care.

When Mrs. Shimada becomes affected with delusions of theft, the caregivers would affirm her reality, and change their response according to Mrs. Shimada's words and actions. Examples include responses such as, "We are keeping it safe for you," "It is safe in your room," or "We will contact the police for you." However, in some cases this would further agitate her. The delusions of theft were causing stress for Mrs. Shimada, and if this situation continued, there was the possibility that her motivation would decline, or her dementia would progress more quickly. In addition, there was a fear that her mental instability would prevent her from maintaining relationships with the staff and other residents.

Therefore, we reviewed our support methods for Mrs. Shimada and switched to Logical Care, in which we firmly conveyed the fact that her niece was taking care of her valuables and encouraged her to accept the fact. Whenever Mrs. Shimada complained that her bankbook was stolen, we told her truthfully that her niece was taking care of her valuables. At the same time, we also asked Mrs. Shimada's family to cooperate, and asked her niece to say "I'm taking care of your valuables" every time she came to visit Mrs. Shimada. As a result of this support, Mrs. Shimada gradually came to accept the facts and regained her composure. Currently, her delusions of theft have almost completely disappeared, and she seems to be leading a calm daily life.

This case indicates the danger of caregivers assuming that a person with dementia is unable to remember facts that are conveyed to them. At the same time, it shows us that with Logical Care, a person with dementia can not only remember old facts, but also acknowledge and accept new facts.

Case 3 Conveying Facts Through Message Cards: Quest to Avoid Physical Restraints

Shigeyuki Sato (pseudonym), age 80, was becoming very forgetful so he entered an elder care facility with his wife. The wife also had dementia, although not to the degree of Mr. Sato. Once they entered the facility, Mr. Sato's condition worsened. He would try to escape the facility and became verbally abusive and violent towards the staff. He was admitted to a psychiatric hospital for medical care and protection and had to leave the elder care facility. Mr. Sato's family consulted with us since he had nowhere to go after being released from the hospital, and it was decided that he and his wife would move to Housenka. Mr. Sato's dementia was at Stage 4 according to Housenka's dementia progression chart.

Even after moving into Housenka, there were times when he would wander, say incoherent things, and become agitated. However, by accepting his behavior and listening to him politely, his tendency for verbal abuse or violence was eliminated. While he still had some anxiety, he was living peacefully. After about three and a half years after moving in, Mr. Sato would often have difficulty swallowing food, and upon examination, advanced esophageal cancer was found.

Since there was a possibility that he would not be able to eat or drink in the future, he was admitted to a hospital for treatment, but Mr. Sato was unable to assess his own situation. He would stubbornly ask why he was there and ask to go home and pull out the IV needle or try to leave the hospital room. Hospital nurses and Housenka caregivers would explain that he was at the hospital to receive treatment for his illness, but he could not understand no matter how many times it was explained. Since there was a risk of not only his condition worsening, but also risks of falling, tripping, or escaping, the hospital decided that physical restraints were necessary.

However, unlike temporary restraints, such as after surgery, restraints that bind residents to a bed can cause unimaginable stress. It may even worsen cognitive symptoms. We believe that restraints should be avoided as much as possible, so we decided to try every conceivable method we could think of, and we decided to try conveying information visually.

We handwrote messages such as "This is a hospital. We are treating your illness," "We are giving you an IV to help you get better (with a picture of an IV)," "Let's get better as soon as possible and go home," on a piece of paper on the spot, had Mr. Sato read them and displayed them in a visible location. This method was apparently very helpful for Mr. Sato. He was able to accept that he was sick and received treatment within one or two hours. In just that short time, Mr. Sato calmed down and accepted the facts. He stopped trying to remove the IV and was able to calmly receive treatment.

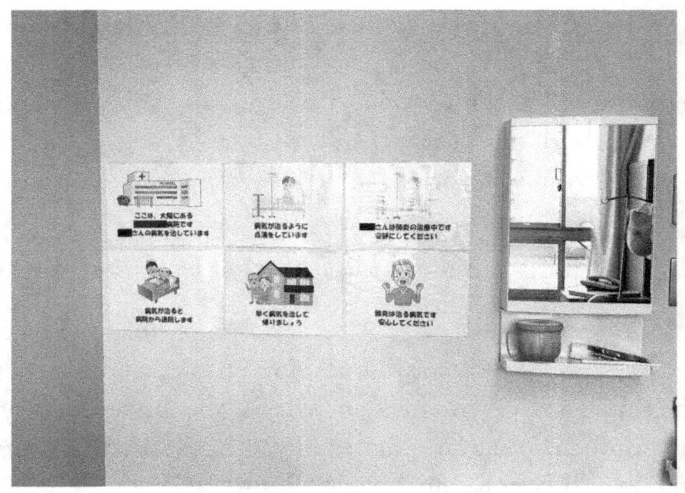

Post message cards in easy-to-see locations.

Of course, this method is not permanent so even if he understood at the time, he would forget again. However, by repeatedly showing him the cards and asking him to read them each time, he became more accepting of the facts, and he was able to stay relatively calm and relaxed during his hospitalization. The handwritten message cards were recreated to be clearer when Mr. Sato's condition calmed down a bit. This case is an example that shows that Logical Care can be easily established through the use of visual methods.

Due to his failing memory, Mr. Sato still asked where he was or what a certain item (such as an IV) was or would walk to the hospital room door several times afterwards. With the cooperation of the hospital nurses, we would show him the message card posted on the wall each time to continue supporting his understanding. As a result, he was able to be treated without physical restraints. Because he had terminal cancer, he passed away about two months after being hospitalized, but I believe that the fact that he was able to live out his final days peacefully helped raise the overall level of happiness in Mr. Sato's life.

The highest priority of a hospital is treatment, and many believe that physical restraints are unavoidable in the name of treatment. However, as mentioned above, this can lead to a vicious cycle of unrest, violence, worsening dementia, prolonged use of physical restraints, and heavy medications. We, as professional caregivers, can contribute to avoiding this negative spiral and protecting a person's dignity. In this case, the hospital agreed with our proposal and cooperated with us. We were able to reach this outcome by working in unison with the medical institution.

Case 4 Visualizing Schedules: Creativity to Ease Anxiety

Kinuko Saeki (pseudonym), age 92, was a resident of Housenka whose dementia was at Stage 4 according to Housenka's dementia progression chart. She would go live with her daughter for about a week every month, so she was probably unaware that she lived in Housenka. Every night, she would say, "This is not my home so I must go home. When can I go home?" and start packing all her clothes. It was also pointed out by her daughter that it was not hygienic since Mrs. Saeki could not distinguish between clean and dirty clothes and pack them all together.

She was unable to understand verbal explanations such as, "You will be going to your daughter's house in three days," or "Separate clothing that needs to be washed." We noticed that Mrs. Saeki would often read books, which meant that her reading comprehension ability was still high. We therefore decided to support her understanding through Logical Care, by structuring her environment to convey facts.

We believed that Mrs. Saeki's anxiety was a result of her not knowing when she would be able to go home. We decided that she would be able to spend the time at Housenka calmly if we eliminated her anxiety by visualizing her schedule and helping her understand it. Specifically, we placed a desk calendar on Mrs. Saeki's desk in her room and wrote down the days she is leaving Housenka and other plans so she could read them. As a result, she was able to understand that there are days when she returns home but she is at Housenka the rest of the days and stopped complaining about wanting to go home. When we explained our care method to the daughter, she was extremely pleased and started to write down the plans on the calendar herself. We also placed a laundry basket in Mrs. Saeki's room and posted a sign that read "Please put underwear and pajamas that need to be washed in here." Once this measure was implemented, Mrs. Saeki would put her own clothes in the laundry basket, without mixing up clean and dirty clothes.

This case shows that presenting and structuring information in an easy-to-understand manner as a means to implement Logical Care led to a creation of a safe environment where Mrs. Saeki can live while drawing out her full potential.

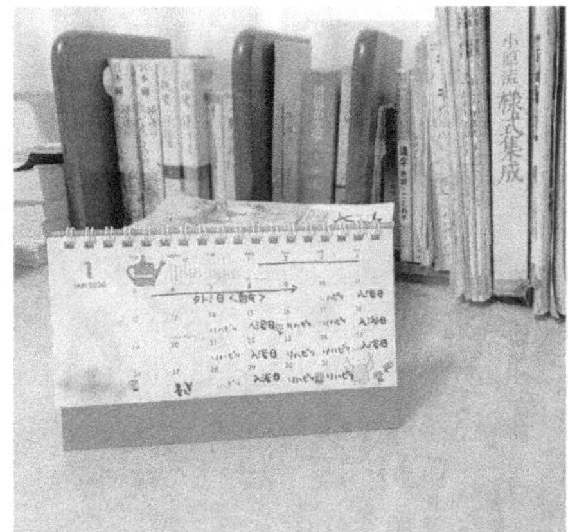

Inscribed plans in a desk calendar

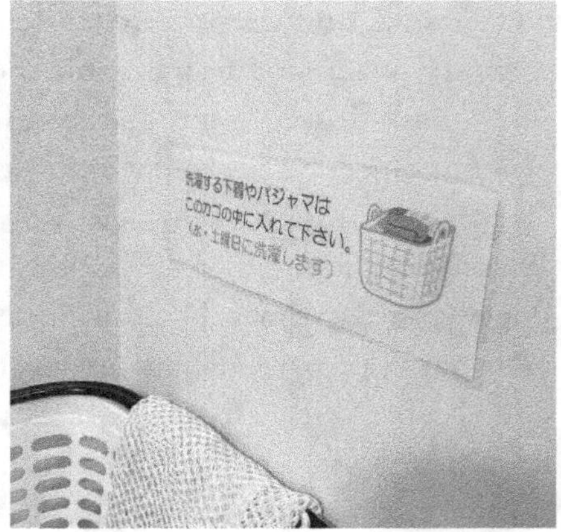

A laundry basket and a posted sign

Case 5 Controlling Inappropriate Sexual Behavior: Help Regain Interest in Hobbies

Eisuke Watanabe (pseudonym), age 70, developed dementia from frontotemporal lobar degeneration (FTLD). His dementia was at Stage 3 according to Housenka's dementia progression chart. Mr. Watanabe was diagnosed with depression while working at a company and retired early. After retiring, he lived a life where he enjoyed his hobbies and other activities but began to exhibit inappropriate sexual behavior in his late 60s. He was warned by the police after making sexual advances toward a woman during a walk and was banned from an adult day care service because he made excessive advances toward female staff and other participants. (As explained in Chapter 1, one of the characteristics of frontotemporal dementia [FTD] is inappropriate sexual behavior. In hindsight, it is obvious that Mr. Watanabe's symptoms were due to FTD, but unfortunately, he was not diagnosed with dementia at the time.)

Mr. Watanabe's wife tried looking for a new adult day care service since she could not watch over her husband at home alone, but her application was rejected by dozens of services. When Mrs. Watanabe took her eyes off of her husband for a few moments, Mr. Watanabe ventured outside and tried to flirt with a woman on the street. The police were called, and they apprehended Mr. Watanabe. His wife explained that Mr. Watanabe was ill, and the woman accepted the explanation, so he was released immediately. However, it was determined that Mr. Watanabe needed treatment and was admitted to a psychiatric hospital.

Mrs. Watanabe realized that she could no longer care for Mr. Watanabe at home, and desperately searched for a residential care facility, but was turned down by 45 facilities because of his inappropriate sexual behavior. The care manager even told her, "There are no facilities that will accept your husband." Mr. Watanabe was permitted to stay in the hospital for a while longer, but his family wanted him to be in a close-to-normal environment to live a more stimulating and motivated life as soon as possible, so they continued to gather information. It was during this time that they learned of Housenka, read my book *Dementia Innovation*, and wrote to us. The family told us that they thought of us as a last resort.

The letter clearly described Mr. Watanabe's uncontrollable sexual desires, including viewing pornographic videos constantly and attempting to invite prostitutes to his home. We could tell from the letter that the family was exhausted and emotionally distressed. Once we received the letter, a group of professionals, including the facility director, doctors, nurses, caregivers, lifestyle consultants, and elder care support specialists, discussed whether Housenka would accept Mr. Watanabe. After considering many factors, we decided to welcome him to Housenka.

The biggest issue was to control his inappropriate sexual behaviors. We had to anticipate the possibility of sexual advances and behavior toward female residents and caregivers and consider measures to respond to them. We also needed to understand FTLD and to work with cooperating physicians to ensure appropriate responses. The physician that diagnosed Mr. Watanabe with FTLD advised us to take precautions in providing care, such as keeping female staff away from the resident as much as possible and finding other interests to replace his sexual interests.

To begin, we decided that Mr. Watanabe would, in principle, be cared for by male caregivers. The caregivers persistently informed him that sexual comments are not allowed, and with the cooperation of his wife, we made sure that there were no discrepancies in the explanations to Mr. Watanabe given to him by his wife or the caregivers.

After establishing such a system, we proceeded to provide concrete support based mostly on Logical Care. The first issue was to shift his interest from sex to other subjects. We knew that Mr. Watanabe liked physical activities and used to play golf when he was younger. We had him experience bo soccer (stick soccer)—a sport where 11-member teams sit in one row across from the opposing team and hit a ball with a stick to try to score a goal. A short time after Mr. Watanabe moved in, there was a stick soccer tournament at the facility, and he scored a goal to excite the crowd. He became completely absorbed in stick soccer after this. Since his interest shifted to something else, we have not seen him engage in inappropriate sexual behavior after moving into Housenka.

In addition to stick soccer, we believe that the care was successful since we structured Mr. Watanabe's lifestyle by creating detailed schedules with his understanding. Too much free time can lead to poor use of time and thinking about interests and desires. In Mr. Watanabe's case, there was concern that his interests would turn toward sexual matters. Therefore, we made a clear schedule for his daily life to create routines for different times of the day. This was another way to prevent him from focusing on sexual matters.

Another measure was to clearly define the placement of watches, glasses, and cellphones, and the like since Mr. Watanabe had particular insistence on their location. This information was shared among our caregivers. This was done to create a space that suited his preferences as much as possible, and to ensure that he could spend time in a stress-free environment.

Through the above Logical Care, Mr. Watanabe's inappropriate sexual behavior—which had been a problem for a long time—was resolved after moving into Housenka, and he has been able to live a calm and peaceful life. Before moving into Housenka, Mrs. Watanabe would be the only one talking when they had a "conversation." However, now, Mr. Watanabe would start the conversation by talking about stick soccer, snacks and the like when he talks to his wife on the phone, which makes Mrs. Watanabe very happy. Mrs. Watanabe said that since her husband moved into Housenka, she has been able to sleep better. Mrs. Watanabe told us that the dramatic improvement in his sexual behavior was like watching a wizard work magic. This case shows that depending on the type of dementia and their condition, telling a person with dementia that "what is good is good and what is bad is bad" and encouraging them to understand can make a big difference in the situation.

In general, affirming the behaviors of the person is important in dementia care. However, behaviors that cause inconvenience to others, endanger their own lives, or unhygienic behaviors, such as incontinence, will ultimately have a negative impact on the person's life. Therefore, in cases such as these, it is important to conduct measures that aim to shift their interest in a different direction.

Finally, we would like to share an excerpt of a letter we received from Mrs. Watanabe a little while after welcoming Mr. Watanabe to Housenka.

"A drowning man will clutch at a straw," is the perfect idiom to describe my situation when I first contacted Housenka. Based on my previous attempts to find a residential care facility, I had completely fallen into the mindset that the facility will listen to my story but end up turning me away anyway. Although I didn't have any hope when I called, I prepared as usual, thinking that it was courtesy to be honest and let you know the truth since you are taking time to listen to me.

"First, I would like to express my appreciation to Ms. Ogura for listening to my long story until the end with sincerity. This action alone eased me a bit and made me think, "I can accept it even if I am rejected again." At the time, I was also providing care to my mother-in-law, so I was mentally exhausted. Even when I attended dementia family meetings, I felt alone because there was no one else who had to deal with handling inappropriate sexual behavior like me. When others would share stories of their burdens of care, I would cynically think that their issues were nothing compared to mine since they didn't have to deal with the police multiple times. No matter how much I searched through books, websites, and the like, I couldn't even find hints about how to deal with my husband's condition. But I sensed those hints in *Dementia Innovation*, as well as in the words of Ms. Ogura and Ms. Nishiwaki.

"I believe there are many families who are too tired to take the initial step in sharing their experience. Or maybe, it may be the Japanese tendency to be modest. I still have the energy and desire to progress step by step. That is why I have decided to have my experience published in some form in the family meeting booklet. There is no textbook on how a family should handle those with frontotemporal lobar degeneration who conduct inappropriate sexual behaviors. This is why my experience with my husband should be left as an example for future use. I would like to express my deepest gratitude to Ms. Ogura, Ms. Nishiwaki, and the other staff of Housenka who saved me from the depths of despair."

We hope that these cases have given you a better understanding of what Logical Care is and how it is practiced in the field. In the next chapter, we will explain and provide case studies of Lateral Care.

Chapter 4
Practical Tips for Lateral Care

Provide Care based on the Person's "Reality"

Care Appropriate for the Situation or Moment

In this chapter, we will explain Lateral Care (Reality Affirmation-Based Aid) in more detail. "Lateral" can mean many things such as "from the side" or "horizontal." In terms of lateral thinking, which is the act of viewing issues from various angles without being bound by stereotypes or fixed notions, it refers to thinking in a horizontal manner that is not only sequentially (vertical thinking). By fusing the concept of lateral thinking with dementia care, we created Lateral Care.

As explained previously, Logical Care (Fact Acceptance-Based Aid) provides care by trying to connect the thoughts of residents and individual situations in a single logical manner. It is when the resident's thoughts, conditions, concept of time or the like constantly seem to drift illogically that Lateral Care, in which caregivers provide care by stepping into the resident's "world," comes into play. To put it simply, Lateral Care provides care that is appropriate for the current situation (or even for individual moments).

In general, "reality" is the "facts" that are currently in front of us, or mental reconstructions of "facts" we have observed. However, the word "reality" in Lateral Care refers to "what the person perceives as reality in their minds." As memory and comprehension deteriorate due to dementia, disorientation, which causes a person to become confused about the current time or location, becomes more common. As a result, they often become confused about the current year and act under the belief that events in their memories are current events. They will try to interpret the situation and people around them according to values of the past. In other words, past memories become the "reality" of the present. Studies show that people often revert to times when they felt accomplishment, such as when they were growing their business venture, when their career was taking off, or when they were working hard to raise their children.

Channel Into the Person's "Reality"

For Lateral Care, caregivers must first accept the current "reality" of the person with dementia. Caregivers must quickly determine the "reality" of each individual situation based on advance assessments and the like and provide care by tuning into that "reality." Instead of denying the "reality," caregivers must accept it in a positive manner and enter that "reality" to provide appropriate care according to the situation.

For example, there was a case of a female resident who would reject bathing. After providing Lateral Care, she would bathe without any issues. This woman hated bathing, especially washing her hair. When caregivers told her that bathing would be refreshing, she would deny it and refuse to bathe. When we were reviewing the care provided to her, we noticed that she would regularly act and speak as if she was working. We asked her family about this and found out that the woman used to own a boutique, and she would always shower, apply makeup, and dress up when going out or meeting people. Using this information, all caregivers were informed to tell her "You are going out now, so you have to shower and wash your hair," when it was time to bathe. Just by changing the phrasing, bathing was no longer an issue. As this case shows, the essence of Lateral Care is for caregivers to tune in and become a part of the person's world to provide care.

Lateral Care Helps Regain Cheerfulness and Vitality

In fact, the care provided to Tamae Yamamoto (pseudonym), whom we have mentioned many times already, was Lateral Care. To briefly review, Mrs. Yamamoto would leave her room at night and start sleeping on the sofa in the common area, so we initially guided her back to her room by telling her negative aspects of sleeping on a sofa. However, continuing to deny Mrs. Yamamoto's behavior caused her to lose vitality and worsen her dementia. Therefore, we decided to review Mrs. Yamamoto's life history, and we interviewed her family again to obtain a detailed understanding of her life history.

From this review, we learned that when Mrs. Yamamoto was a nurse, she worked many night shifts and usually took a nap on the sofa during that time. If Mrs. Yamamoto's current "reality" is that she is still a nurse, then sleeping on the sofa would be more natural for her than sleeping on the bed in her room. Once we let her sleep on the sofa, we could tell by her facial expressions and posture when she was sleeping that she was more comfortable, and we realized that sleeping on the sofa is "reality that comes naturally" for Mrs. Yamamoto. This event led us to switch to Lateral Care, to provide care that affirms Mrs. Yamamoto's "reality" and is based on her thoughts and actions, so that she can live a comfortable life. As a result, Mrs. Yamamoto slept soundly on the sofa, woke up refreshed in the morning, and most importantly, she seemed more at peace.

Other actions, such as standing closely and listening carefully to caregivers when they are conducting a handover or taking vital signs, also showed that Mrs. Yamamoto is a nurse in her "reality." These actions are just like an experienced nurse gently instructing rookie nurses. She would even often look after other residents, further signaling her nurse mindset. We accept Mrs. Yamamoto's "reality" of being a nurse and ask her to push other residents' wheelchairs when they move as a group to fulfill her sense of duty and responsibility. This simple action of responsibly pushing a "patient's" wheelchair causes Mrs. Yamamoto to smile. Through Lateral Care, Mrs. Yamamoto was able to regain cheerfulness and vitality.

To a Person With Dementia, Everything is "Reality"

Next, we will explain the key points to conducting Lateral Care. Before accepting a resident's "reality" and becoming part of it to provide care, we must first determine what that resident's "reality" is. As previously mentioned, people with disorientation often have difficulty forecasting future events and instead revert to a mindset of past personal experiences. For this reason, it is important to have a thorough understanding of a resident's life history through interviews with the resident and their families.

As explained in the section "Determine the Appropriate Method for the Person Through Assessment" (see pg. 116), Housenka also enters information such as common behaviors, remarks, and facial expressions, frequented locations within the facility, people who often appear in conversation, compatibility with other residents, and monikers that the resident responds well to in the assessment sheet and use this information to better understand the resident's current worldview. Based on this information, we then observe the resident's words and actions and think about what age the resident is, the times they are living in and other backgrounds that may be true in their "reality." Once we are able to determine the resident's current "reality," we are able to tune into that reality and become part of it to better provide care.

For example, there was a resident who became restless in the evening. Upon closer observation, it appeared that she was getting ready to pick someone up. When we asked her daughter about it, she told us that her mother would always pick her up from cram school ever since she was young. From this fact we can hypothesize that the resident is currently living in a reality where she is still busy from child rearing, and she is trying to go pick up her daughter every evening. These small clues help us determine the individual "realities" that we must tune into to provide appropriate care.

An important point when determining the current "reality" is to see the resident's response to names, monikers, and the like that they were addressed by in the past. When repeating this trial-and-error process, in addition to monitoring whether or not they respond, it is important to monitor how responses change depending on different tone of voice (male or female tone), names addressed by, body language and the like. In the next section, we will introduce some case studies of Lateral Care.

Lateral Care Case Studies

Case 1 Hiding Facts to Fit the Worldview: For a Peaceful Death

Takashi Sasaki (pseudonym), age 96, lost his wife when he was 91 and his son to illness when he was 94. When his son passed away, Mr. Sasaki experienced health problems, and due to the progression of dementia, he would constantly forget about the death of his son, so he was unable to recognize the fact. His family could no longer take care of him at home due to advanced dementia, so he entered Housenka. When he entered, worried about Mr. Sasaki's health, the widow of his son asked us to hide the fact that the son passed away and instead tell him that his son is hospitalized for an illness. Mr. Sasaki's dementia was at Stage 5 according to Housenka's dementia progression chart.

Mr. Sasaki quickly showed a strong desire to return home after entering Housenka, and he often appeared restless and hyperactive. He would constantly express concern about his son. Each time, the caregiver would explain that his son is in a nearby hospital so not to worry. Mr. Sasaki could see the lobby on the first floor from the floor where his room was, and every evening, he would see somebody leaving from the lobby. We hypothesized that this environment was increasing his desire to return home, and reminded him of his children who are home, which may have amplified his concern for the son, who he thought was in the hospital. We switched Mr. Sasaki's floor to one where the lobby was not visible, which led to him expressing a desire to return home less frequently. However, he still regularly expressed his desires to return home and see his son.

Based on this situation, we did not believe it was wise to inform Mr. Sasaki of his son's death, so we had to seek new ways to support him in an effort to somehow alleviate his stress. When we observed Mr. Sasaki's behavior closely, we noticed that there were often times where he did not know what to do due to the unfamiliar environment. Close observation revealed that he was spending much of his time idle due to his unfamiliarity with his environment. Therefore, we decided to test out care that steers a person away from negative thoughts by providing a relaxing environment where they can enjoy hobbies and the like.

At Housenka, the board game *Go* is played as part of recreational activities. We observed that Mr. Sasaki would concentrate for hours when he played *Go*. So, we asked for the cooperation of other residents and increased opportunities to enjoy *Go*. To be honest, we were worried whether or not Mr. Sasaki still understood the rules since his dementia was very advanced. However, our worries turned out to be unfounded. Not only did he understand the rules fully, but his play would also result in intense games that drew crowds. We believe that playing *Go* helped alleviate Mr. Sasaki's loneliness and anxiety from moving to a new environment, and the attention he received created a comfortable atmosphere that helped him to develop a sense of camaraderie. He would still ask where he was at times, but he would seem satisfied when told that it was a place to play *Go*.

Another meeting with Mr. Sasaki's family was held, and it was reaffirmed that the news of his son's death would be kept hidden due to concerns about Mr. Sasaki's mental and physical health. We provided Lateral Care by affirming Mr. Sasaki's worldview that his son was still alive, and whenever he brought up his son, we responded as if the son was still alive. Mr. Sasaki passed away due to old age about five months after entering Housenka, but he was able to live a peaceful and comfortable life during his last moments. His family also expressed their relief and gratitude, saying they were grateful that Mr. Sasaki was able to spend his last days peacefully and without grief.

Some may say that continuing to lie about his son's death is not the right thing to do. To be honest, there were conflicting opinions even amongst our caregivers. However, after comprehensively considering that 1) Mr. Sasaki fell ill the first time he learned of his son's death, 2) the strong desire of the family to keep it a secret, and 3) his physical deterioration due to his advanced age, we decided to provide Lateral Care by affirming a "reality" that Mr. Sasaki accepts—one where his son is still alive.

I personally believe that there is no major benefit in forcefully making a person nearing the last stages of life to accept a harsh reality.

Since the primary goal of care is for the individual to live peacefully and comfortably, we did not see the merit in providing Logical Care (Fact Acceptance-Based Aid) in this case. On the other hand, in the case of Eiko Ueyama (pseudonym), who was tricked into entering Housenka (see Chapter 3), we changed our method from Lateral Care to Logical Care because we judged that it was necessary for Mrs. Ueyama to lead a stable life at Housenka. We also evaluated Mrs. Ueyama's condition, personality, and the like, and judged that she would be able to accept facts if they were conveyed to her honestly.

To what extent should facts be conveyed to a person with dementia? There is no one, simple answer. It is a case-by-case process, and the decision should be made carefully based on what is best for the individual with consideration to the family's desires.

Case 2 Pretending to Be Family Members: Massive Improvement in Denial of Care

Yoshimi Endo (pseudonym) aged 67, had symptoms of disorientation such as not knowing where she was even when near her own home. She would also often scrape or bump her car when driving. Her family contacted Housenka after Mrs. Endo was diagnosed with Alzheimer's disease at age 63 and it became difficult for her to safely live at home. However, Mrs. Endo stubbornly refused to move in, so we asked her to try having meals and haircuts at the restaurant and salon at Housenka to get used to the environment first. Her time at Housenka was gradually increased, and she moved in after she became accustomed to the atmosphere, nine months after the initial consultation. Mrs. Endo's dementia was at Stage 6 according to Housenka's dementia progression chart.

After moving in, Mrs. Endo was very emotional, had sudden mood swings, and was verbally abusive and violent toward other residents and our caregivers. She would also refuse to bathe and keep herself clean. We suspected that these issues were due to the stress caused by communication issues between us and Mrs. Endo. Another behavior we noticed was that, perhaps because she and her husband ran a company together, she seemed to think that male caregivers were her employees and men in suits were business partners. She also thought that female caregivers were her brother's wife, who was the one who mainly took care of Mrs. Endo after she developed dementia. In addition, she thought that certain caregivers were her husband or daughter, and she would regularly have friendly conversations with them.

At first, Logical Care was provided, so when Mrs. Endo called those caregivers by her husband or daughter's name, they corrected her and stated their actual names. However, we noticed that this would make her grumpy. After discussion with her family, we decided to switch to Lateral Care to provide care by having the caregivers pretend to be the roles that Mrs. Endo has given them in her "reality." The caregivers other than the ones pretending to be family members also started to refer to Mrs. Endo as "President Endo," which was how she was called when she ran her company. She responded much better when addressed as such. In addition, we observed that Mrs. Endo must have had deep trust in her husband. She would regularly ask the caregiver who was her "husband" about what to do. The "husband" would talk to her gently and ask her to do things that connect to care. Mrs. Endo was also particular about how people spoke to her. Her expression would become grim especially when a woman with a high-pitched voice spoke quickly. The "husband" tried to mimic the actual husband's speech patterns as much as possible by changing how fast he spoke and his voice tone. The family has also noted how Mrs. Endo's hearing seems better and more sensitive after developing dementia (also see Article #3: Sensory Changes Caused by dementia on page 86).

Having caregivers pretend to be her family improved the relationship between us and Mrs. Endo. The bathing process became less of a burden when her "family" provided bathing assistance. Furthermore, we discovered that Mrs. Endo does not like to have water splashed on her face, so we began to use a towel to protect her face while bathing. Combined with adjusting the water temperature to a lower setting to fit Mrs. Endo's preference, these measures increased the number of baths from about 15 times a month to 25 times a month.

The quality of communication also improved drastically as a result of increasing opportunities for Mrs. Endo to talk with residents she is close with during daytime activities, as well as using a separate personalized service to have her enjoy conversing while taking a walk. These various measures helped Mrs. Endo calm down. This is proven by the fact that the number of violent episodes, which was about 14 times a month before measures were implemented, dropped significantly to three times in the three months after measures were implemented.

This case reiterated the importance of thoroughly understanding a resident's life history, preferences, and the like to correctly tune into their current "reality."

Case 3 Playing the Roles Desired in the World of the Person With Dementia

Hisao Sugawara, age 84, a former restaurant owner, always liked drinking but his alcohol consumption increased significantly when he had family issues. He was diagnosed with alcoholic dementia after turning 80, and moved into Housenka when he began to exhibit inappropriate behaviors such as walking around the common area of his apartment naked. Mr. Sugawara's dementia was at Stage 6 according to Housenka's dementia progression chart.

When he entered Housenka, his "reality" was that he was still working hard managing a restaurant, and believed that our caregivers were employees, accountants, or important business partners. We could have ignored his "reality" or informed him of the "fact" that he is no longer a restaurant owner. However, to do so is to disaffirm Mr. Sugawara and his inability to accept "facts," which can rob him of his vitality and worsen his cognitive symptoms. Therefore, we decided to provide Lateral Care by stepping into Mr. Sugawara's "reality" and playing the roles he believes to be true.

For example, when he asks the caregiver (who is the "accountant") about transferring money, the "accountant" would reply that they already made the transfer, which would please Mr. Sugawara greatly. He would bow deeply and talk politely when speaking to the "important business partner" while he would relentlessly use harsh words to his "employees."

If this situation arose before Housenka adapted Lateral Care, the caregivers who were subject to the harsh words would not have thought of understanding Mr. Sugawara's "reality." Even if they understand that Mr. Sugawara's actions are caused by dementia, they might still feel that their work is hard and unrewarding, which can lead to stress or even depression. However, now that Lateral Care has been introduced, our caregivers know that they must become actors at times to implement it correctly. In this case, the "employees" would actively play the role of Mr. Sugawara's preferred employees. We believe that having our caregivers understand the concepts of Lateral Care and putting it into practice has allowed them to learn about the "realities" of people with dementia and provide care in a more relaxed and enjoyable manner.

Switching to Lateral Care also brought positive changes to the relationships between Mr. Sugawara and his family. When we were discussing the switch to Lateral Care with Mrs. Sugawara, she informed us that there were times when her husband could not recognize her. She agreed to act normally as his wife if Mr. Sugawara recognized her, and act like a stranger when he could not recognize her. This is something I also personally experienced when my beloved grandmother developed dementia, so I understand that the shock of being forgotten by a loved one cannot be explained by words. However, Mrs. Sugawara accepted the situation and helped provide support by also tuning into Mr. Sugawara's "reality."

Before Mr. Sugawara moved into Housenka, Mrs. Sugawara tried to go along with Mr. Sugawara's inconsistent stories, but she would get scolded when she failed to do so. This confused and exhausted her, and along with the devastation of witnessing her husband walk around the common area naked, she would often find herself in tears. Since Mr. Sugawara moved into Housenka, Mrs. Sugawara has been able to live peacefully. She also realized that our care resulted in peaceful expressions by Mr. Sugawara, so she agreed to also respond in such ways.

When taking care of a person with dementia at home, communication issues between that person and the caregiver can cause relationships to become tense or even fall apart. In the above case, moving into Housenka created some much-needed distance between the husband and wife, and with the support of care professionals, they were able to return to a relationship where they can share a laugh. We believe that this rewarding scene of repaired relationships is an outcome of Lateral Care.

Case 4 Supporting Desires: To Maintain Sense of Purpose and Vitality

Takashi Onodera, age 67, who had early-onset dementia, was being cared for at home by his family, and used the short-stay program at Housenka. However, as his dementia progressed, he often became paranoid and exhibited dangerous behavior such as violence towards his family, so he was moved to Housenka full time. Mr. Onodera's dementia was at Stage 6 according to Housenka's dementia progression chart. Mr. Onodera would wander even while he was using our short-stay program, and this behavior continued when he moved in. When he was at Housenka for the short-stay program, we stopped his wandering since it could have led to unnecessary trouble (such as accidentally entering someone else's room). Mr. Onodera would have a displeased expression when we stopped his wandering. After Mr. Onodera moved in, we decided to observe his wandering more carefully. He would wander throughout the day, but he would have a relaxed expression, as if he was enjoying a stroll.

In many cases, people with dementia who are wandering will have a stern expression. This is a sign that the person is wandering due to stress, and it should be stopped. However, we concluded that stopping the wandering of someone who seems relaxed and comfortable while wandering, like Mr. Onodera, could lead to greater stress. The displeased expression Mr. Onodera would show when we stopped his wandering is proof of this. Additionally, many recent studies show the benefits that walking has on the body and brain. Although we do not know the "reality" that Mr. Onodera is living while wandering, after considering these factors, we decided to affirm his desire to walk and let him walk as much as he likes.

When we asked him to wear a pedometer, we found out that Mr. Onodera would walk around 40,000 steps on some days. Before gaining this information, when Mr. Onodera told us that he was hungry, we would assume he forgot that he already ate due to dementia and provide candy or the like. But seeing the amount he walks, there was no way that the 1,600-calorie diet prepared for the elderly residents each day would be sufficient. We consulted with a nutritionist and decided to support Mr. Onodera's desire to walk from the dietary aspect as well, for example, by making his serving of rice larger or adding milk. When we informed the family of this change, they began to cooperate without hesitation, such as by bringing snacks or rice balls when they visited, and walking together and conversing as he wandered as if it was a normal stroll. In addition to walking, Mr. Onodera also liked to swim. One day, he let out a cheerful yell, jumped into the bathtub and started swimming. Since then, we adjust his bath time, so that he does not disturb other residents, and let him swim as much as he likes while caregivers are watching over him.

Under conventional dementia care, the main issues for Mr. Onodera's case would be "how to reduce wandering" or "what is the cause of wandering." However, under our Lateral Care, we let him wander since it was relaxing for him and also supported him through dietary and other means so he can walk as much as he likes. This case shows that aspect of Lateral Care that tries to support the person's "will to live" as much as possible, as long as it is not dangerous or causing pain.

Case 5 Controlling Temperament Through Singing and Care by Supporting Friendships

Tae Kawasaki (pseudonym), age 86, gradually began to dislike cooking, which she had always enjoyed, after turning 80, and was diagnosed with Dementia with Lewy Bodies (DLB) when she visited a clinic. She entered a residential home for elders but transferred to Housenka when her dementia progressed. Mrs. Kawasaki's dementia was at Stage 5 according to Housenka's dementia progression chart.

A major issue when caring for people with dementia is the difficulty communicating. This was the case for Mrs. Kawashima. She was very temperamental and relatively calm when she was in a good mood, but when something suddenly angered her, she became inaccessible and could not be cared for. She would respond when someone called her name but did not seem to understand subsequent conversations and the like. She would show signs of rejection, but we were unable to understand what Mrs. Kawashima was saying, leading to even more difficulty communicating. She would also speak to the mirror in a language no one could understand and became angry when her reflection did not respond. This is a symptom called mirror phenomenon, which appears as part of core symptoms of aphasia and disorientation.

Mrs. Kawashima also refused assistance with bathing and toileting, and often urinated and defecated in common areas such as hallways and dining rooms, as well as in other residents' rooms. She could not understand pictograms that clearly indicated the location of toilets. We needed to think of countermeasures quickly, since this situation might lead to hygiene problems or trouble with other residents. However, since we could not communicate with Mrs. Kawashima through speaking or writing, first we needed to figure out what affected her mood and how to keep her in a good mood.

Our first attempt was to modify how we spoke to Mrs. Kawashima. We thought that perhaps increasing the number of times the caregivers spoke to her while also providing more detail may help improve verbal communication. For example, to provide better toileting assistance, we regularly asked her if she needed to go to the toilet, in addition to observing when she left the dining rooms after meals and setting up sensor mats near her bed, to better monitor her behavior throughout the day. When she actually went to the toilet, we would explain every step, such as by saying, "I am pulling down your pants now," and check Mrs. Kawashima's response before assisting. These measures occasionally worked if the caregiver was able to lead Mrs. Kawashima to the toilet when she actually needed to go, but the outcomes were not sufficient, and it did not solve her temperamental issues.

When our caregivers were discussing Mrs. Kawashima's behavior with each other, one of them suggested that we can use her facial expressions and emotions as criteria to determine whether or not she understands what is being said. The caregiver reported that upon observation, he noticed that Mrs. Kawashima would hum a Hawaiian tune at times, which seemed to indicate that she was in a good mood. After this discussion, a caregiver imitated Mrs. Kawashima's humming in her presence, and it clearly improved her mood. We decided to nod at what Mrs. Kawashima is saying and speak to her normally if she is in a good mood even if she does not seem to understand. If she is in a bad mood, a caregiver would first hum the Hawaiian tune, and provide care only after her expression relaxes. Using this approach, Mrs. Kawashima was able to communicate with us not verbally, but through emotions and facial expressions based on moods.

Next, our assessment revealed that one of the few phrases of Mrs. Kawashima's that was comprehensible and that she often said was "I have to clean up." Based on this information, we asked her to do some simple cleaning tasks, such as wiping dining room tables, and she would happily complete the task. We would show our appreciation to build a relationship of trust with Mrs. Kawashima. As a result of these efforts, Mrs. Kawashima became less temperamental, and she stopped refusing bathing and toileting assistance. The trust also allowed caregivers to speak to or instruct her at a more appropriate time, which caused her to stop urinating or defecating in inappropriate places.

A little while after Mrs. Kawashima entered Housenka, she made a friend. Yoriko Kubota (pseudonym), age 80, entered Housenka about three months after Mrs. Kawashima. Their conversation sounds like it is in a foreign language that we cannot understand at all, but Mrs. Kubota regularly nods her head to agree with Mrs. Kawashima. Sometimes, they are so focused on their conversation that they forget about mealtimes. It is a textbook example of "being on the same wavelength." These days, they continue to be in each other's presence at all times, creating a magical world filled with fun and peace that has no place for negativity caused by dementia. Perhaps Mrs. Kawashima's rejection of care and irregular bowel movements were caused by the loneliness and anxiety caused by disorientation and aphasia. Now she lives a much calmer life, and enthusiastically wipes the table when we ask her to.

This case illustrates the difficulty of communication when practicing Lateral Care. In a situation where even the professional caregivers had difficulty comprehending Mrs. Kawashima's needs, we attempted to read her facial expressions and emotions to decipher her mood, and through various trial-and-error attempts, we were eventually able to bring about positive change. In addition, gaining Mrs. Kubota as a friend also contributed greatly to improving Mrs. Kawashima's quality of life. The same can be said for Mrs. Kubota.

As caregivers, it is also important for us to assess the compatibility of people with dementia and help them build friendships. Mrs. Kawashima's daughter praised our methods by saying, "my mother was very shy when she was younger, so I still can't believe she made a friend at Housenka and seems so happy talking. This would not have been possible if I was caring for her at home, so I am really glad that she is able to live here."

Care does not function well if it only consists of one-way assistance. Just like in daily life for all people, communication is the key to harmony and enriching the lives of all parties involved. Especially in environments such as an elder care facility where many people live under one roof, it is important to consider how to connect residents with each other. If we can cultivate kindness among residents to help each other, it will greatly improve the atmosphere of a dementia care facility.

Article #3
Sensory Changes Caused by Dementia

Studies show that people's senses become duller as they age, and such a tendency is also seen in many cases described in this book. However, it is interesting to note that instead of becoming dull, there are occasionally people whose senses become so acute or even hypersensitive, as mentioned in "Case 2 Pretending to Be Family Members: Massive Improvement in Denial of Care" in this chapter.

Satoko Suzuki (pseudonym), age 83, a resident of Housenka with Alzheimer's disease, is one of those cases. Mrs. Suzuki's dementia is at Stage 5 according to Housenka's dementia progression chart. Whenever Mrs. Suzuki is in the presence of other residents, such as in the dining room, she is able to hear almost every voice or sound and reacts to all of them. When someone says, "What is this?" she responds, "I wonder what it is," while she might say, "Are you okay?" or "What happened?" when someone says, "Ow." When this happens, she does not face the direction where the voice is coming from. Rather, she continues to face front and responds to the voices by mumbling under her breath. According to her family, Mrs. Suzuki's hearing improved after developing dementia. Indeed, it seemed that her hearing was hypersensitive, and she was overreacting to the voices around her.

Since Mrs. Suzuki is a wheelchair user, she cannot leave an area on her own even if she feels that it is noisy. We decided that it was a huge burden to continue responding to every sound, so we set up an environment where she can privately dine in small groups, such as with her family. We tried to create a quiet place that reduces the amount of information that reaches her ears. As a result, Mrs. Suzuki stopped mumbling and was able to stay calm. Since Mrs. Suzuki has always been a sociable person with many friends, this measure is only taken when she eats. She spends time with other residents during activities and other social gatherings.

In this case, Mrs. Suzuki's life was improved by creating a new living space that can be used at appropriate times to remove stress, instead of just focusing on communication as in Logical Care, Lateral Care, or Integrative Care. Sensory hypersensitivity is also commonly seen in autistic people. Studies show that when information from the ears is overwhelming and causes panic to someone with autism, wearing earmuffs or ear plugs to shut out the information may help to calm them down.

There are also those who experience sensory changes rather than sensory hypersensitivity. The following is also a case about a Housenka resident. One day, he started to complain that the food smelled bad or did not taste good and started to eat less and less. First, we thought that he may have a biased opinion about the food provided at care facilities, so we put his meal in a disposable bento box and told him that it was purchased at a store. However, he would say, "It smells like the food provided here (Housenka)," and refuse to eat. When the doctor made a house call to Housenka, he conducted an olfactory test by asking the resident to sniff a tissue paper soaked in various foods such as soy sauce. The resident responded that the soy sauce smelled like vinegar while the apple smelled like grapes. This series of tests revealed that there was a change in his sense of smell.

Humans enjoy eating not only with our sense of taste but also with our sense of smell. When we cannot smell or perceive different smells, we perceive different flavors even if the food tastes the same. The tests seem to indicate that this person's inability to enjoy food properly was due to an abnormality in his sense of smell.

When he returned home temporarily, he was disappointed when he returned, saying that the food at home tastes different. We conducted various measures to support him, and when we served a meal that had a stronger seasoning than usual, he was finally able to enjoy his meal. His change in sense of smell seemed to be the cause of his change in taste.

In cases such as these, it is possible that dementia is causing sensory changes or hypersensitivity. Caregivers need to act against these symptoms by pursuing the cause of the symptoms and adjusting the environment appropriately. The relationship between dementia and sensory change is a subject that piques the interest of many researchers.

In addition, researchers are interested in the work of Professor Akira Midorikawa of Chuo University, who specializes in clinical neuropsychology, and points out that "sensory hypersensitivity may be one of the causes of behavioral and psychological symptoms of dementia." He is referring to a case in which a previously mild-mannered person became irritated by the voice of his favorite grandchild as his dementia symptoms progressed (reported in "Focusing on Hypersensitivity," *Chuo Online*).

We are also very interested in whether dementia really affects the senses, and if so, what the mechanisms and symptoms are. We hope to continue gaining knowledge and experience in actual care settings to explore this topic.

Chapter 5
Practical Tips for Integrative Care

Fusion of Logical Care and Lateral Care

Flexibly Change the Method of Care

Hopefully, our explanations have given you a better understanding of Logical Care (Fact Acceptance-Based Aid) and Lateral Care (Reality Affirmation-Based Aid). As we have stated many times before, each case of dementia is different. There may be cases in which the person with dementia does not respond well to either Logical Care or Lateral Care. In fact, there have been more than a few such cases at Housenka as well. In such cases, Integrative Care (Comprehensive Aid) will be effective. Rather than applying either Logical Care or Lateral Care, Integrative Care is a method that incorporates the best aspects of both. "Integrative" means combined or united. When there are conflicting ideas for dealing with an individual person or situation, the choice is usually A or B, but Integrative Care strives to search for a solution that combines the best aspects of A and B.

As we were practicing the methods we introduced in *Dementia Innovation*, we have come to understand that dementia symptoms vary depending on the situation and circumstances, even in the same person. For example, a resident receiving Logical Care may be able to understand the facts for certain things but not others, or a resident suited for Lateral Care may be able to accept facts and calm down only in certain situations.

After witnessing these cases, we realized we also needed a method that integrates the best aspects of Logical Care and Lateral Care and applies them fluidly depending on the resident's expressions, actions, and level of understanding for each situation. When we actually implemented this new idea, we found that it was effective. We named this new method

"Integrative Care (Comprehensive Aid)" and decided to introduce it to the world in this book.

Just like the symptoms of dementia, *when* to switch the method of care is different depending on various aspects such as the individual's physical and mental state, the situation, and the time (morning or evening). Caregivers must assess the situation through factors such as how the resident is expressing dissatisfaction or anxiety and how they respond to the actions or words of caregivers, and fluidly switch the method. If communication is possible with the resident, Logical Care may be better, while Lateral Care may be more effective if that resident is in his own "reality." It is important to remember that caregivers cannot force a method onto a situation; simply put, respecting the situation and being empathic helps the resident accept the care and leads to better outcomes.

For us caregivers, events are connected in chronological order, so we tend to subconsciously think that people will understand something that they understood earlier. However, people with dementia may not be inputting and processing information quickly enough, or that information may be processed differently in their brain. Therefore, if we think in terms of our "common sense," issues will arise while providing care. For example, if a caregiver thinks, "Logical Care worked earlier, so I can continue using Logical Care," without assessing the current situation, the resident may show a confused or panicked expression. In this case, the caregiver must quickly switch to Lateral Care.

Do Not Base the Decision on the Severity of Cognitive Symptoms

It is important to note that although it is often thought that Logical Care is appropriate for those with mild cognitive symptoms, Lateral Care for those with severe symptoms, and Integrative Care for those in between, this is not always the case. It is true to some degree that people with milder symptoms tend to have a higher ability to understand and less memory impairment, and can still communicate rather normally, while those with severe symptoms have a higher possibility of becoming immersed in their "reality." However, there are cases when even those with severe symptoms can understand and accept the current situation if it is truthfully conveyed to them. Our dementia care methods are characterized by an approach that is designed to relieve anxiety and promote acceptance in each situation. Since it does not aim to be a universal solution for all aspects of a resident's life, the appropriate care method cannot be decided solely on the basis of the severity of the resident's cognitive symptoms.

Another related point to remember when applying Integrative Care is that one should not assume that Logical Care or Lateral Care always apply in the same situations. Caregivers must not forget that a person with dementia may react in a completely different way even if applying the same care method that was previously effective in the same situation. In other words, the caregiver must be able to instantly infer what is causing a nuisance, the resident's desires, and so on based on the resident's facial expressions, eye movement, degree of tension and the like. To give an extreme example, something minor may change the situation, making it better to switch to Logical Care even if the resident was relaxed due to Lateral Care five minutes ago. Rather than just deciding once and continuing to rigidly apply that method, one needs to be flexible and adaptive by assessing the resident's reactions (facial expressions, behavior, etc.) on the spot.

The following concepts may not be directly related to dementia care, but I believe they are important, because the common thread among our three methods is to develop techniques to establish communication. *In Management: Tasks, Responsibilities, Practices*, Peter Drucker, the father of management defined the fundamentals of communications as follows: 1) Communication is perception, 2) Communication is expectation, 3) Communication makes demands, and 4) Communication and information are different and indeed largely opposite—yet interdependent. He also states, "Communication is the act of the recipient. In communicating, whatever the medium, the first question has to be 'Is this communication within the recipient's range of perception? Can he receive it?' There is no possibility of communication, in other words, unless we first know what the recipient, the true communicator, can see and why." I truly believe that this is how communication in dementia care should strive to be.

Foundation of the Building Blocks for Ultimate Care

Dementia care is not just a science; it also has elements of art. An artistic sense is especially required in Integrative Care, where caregivers must create ways to provide care that is appropriate to the situation. This may make it sound like a difficult method of care, but to put it simply, caregivers are required to be attentive to the feelings of the person with dementia. This is not necessarily a method that is easy to practice just because a professional caregiver has been working in the field for a long time. Some people say that family members can actually practice Integrative Care better than professionals because they know the person well and can discern what is best for the person.

Even if a person's cognitive functions have deteriorated, they often retain many of their abilities to complete activities of daily living (ADL) and the will to live that they have developed over the years. We believe that the ultimate care is one that draws out and supports these instincts to the very end, and Integrative Care is the foundation of the building blocks that will realize the ultimate care for an individual.

In the next section, we will introduce some case studies of Integrative Care.

Integrative Care Case Studies

Case 1 Changing How to Interact Depending on the Situation: For Realization of a Stable Life

Hisayo Haraguchi (pseudonym), age 93, was diagnosed with Alzheimer's disease in her 80's and was using an elder day care service in Hiroshima, where she lived. When she was 89, she fell and started living with her daughter, who lived in Osaka, because she needed nursing care. Her husband passed away that same year. She entered Housenka when she was 90 because the daughter who was taking care of her had a heart attack.

Mrs. Haraguchi's dementia was at Stage 5 according to Housenka's dementia progression chart.

According to her family, Mrs. Haraguchi used to be a top salesperson, and actively demonstrated her leadership skills in the workplace. Perhaps because of this, she seems to think of herself as the boss and our caregivers and the other residents as her subordinates. She often scolded others if she noticed something that bothered her, such as their language, the way they bowed, and dropping crumbs when eating, and had been observed arguing with other residents and trying to hit them with her cane. If this situation continued and relationships with other residents deteriorated, we would have had to restrict her from interacting with other residents, even though it could be bad for Mrs. Haraguchi's health, since she was a naturally talkative person.

No matter how much we explained to her, she would still believe that other residents were her subordinates. As an attempt to reduce conflicts with other residents, we accepted Mrs. Haraguchi's "reality" and placed her at a dining table with those who were less likely to drop crumbs so she would not have to witness behaviors that bothered her. As a result, she began to have fewer incidents with others.

Although one issue was alleviated, Mrs. Haraguchi also expressed strong desires to return home and displayed symptoms of disorientation. She would often say, "Where am I?" "I want to go back to Hiroshima," and "Where is my husband?" If the caregiver did not respond appropriately, she would become restless and unsteady. She also experienced insomnia and wandering at night.

Now, when Mrs. Haraguchi becomes confused about where she is, we tell her the fact that she is living close to her daughter. We also asked the daughter to write a letter that explains that Mrs. Haraguchi is currently in Osaka and show her the letter when she has trouble accepting the situation. However, there are still times when she insists that she is currently in Hiroshima even when we tell her the facts. After some trial and error, we discovered that she would calm down if we responded according to her "reality."

When she is searching for her dead husband, sometimes she understands when the caregiver says, "I'm sorry your husband passed away," while looking at the family photo in her room, but sometimes she would not be able to accept facts and angrily say, "Why would you say something like that?" In such cases, she will calm down if the caregiver says something along the lines of, "I'm sorry, I confused you for someone else. Your husband is at work." In this way, we decided to change how to respond depending on Mrs. Haraguchi's condition. We start off with conveying facts, and if she has a hard time accepting facts, we communicate according to her "reality."

Another issue was that Mrs. Haraguchi often complained of hunger and asked for snacks. We asked her family to place her favorite foods on the shelves and in the refrigerator in her room, but sometimes she was unable to eat them because she could not understand where they were. To solve this issue, we applied Logical Care and posted a sign on the shelf and refrigerator that showed the layout of the food so that she can comprehend the information visually. As a result, she was able to get her favorite snacks on her own.

This is a textbook example of Integrative Care, in which care is provided based on Logical Care, but the individual's reactions are monitored each time to switch to Lateral Care as necessary. This was a case of repeated trial and error for us, as there was difficulty providing care until we were able to find this balance between Logical Care and Lateral Care. By thoroughly implementing a policy among our caregivers to flexibly respond to Mrs. Haraguchi's reactions each time, she was gradually able to relax more often, leading to a stabler life. These days, she enjoys friendly interactions with other residents.

Case 2 Using Pictograms: Dramatic Improvement in Urinary and Fecal Incontinence

This is a case where aspects of Lateral Care were incorporated into structuring, a major method in Logical Care. Tateo Nakagawa (pseudonym), age 80, was a resident whose dementia was at Stage 5 according to Housenka's dementia progression chart. When he just entered Housenka, he was often observed restlessly walking around the floor where his room was located. He would become confused about where he was as he was walking, leading to trouble such as entering other residents' rooms and urinary or fecal incontinence because he could not find the toilet.

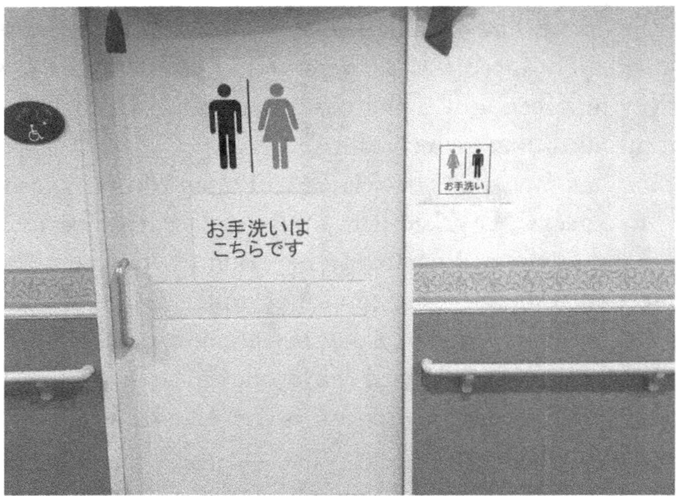

The pictogram posted on the common toilet.

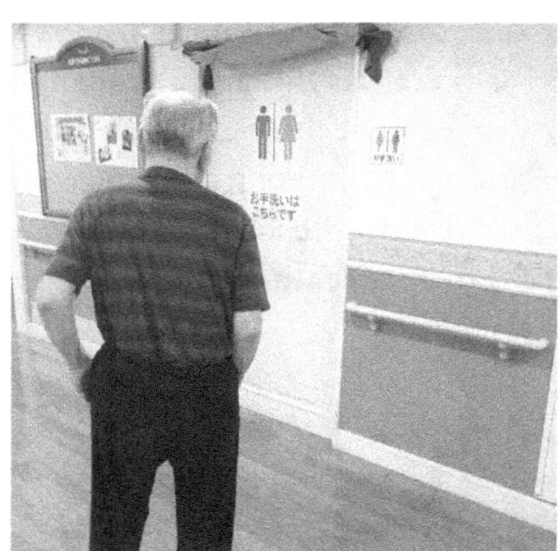

Mr. Nakagawa sees the pictogram and heads to the toilet on his own.

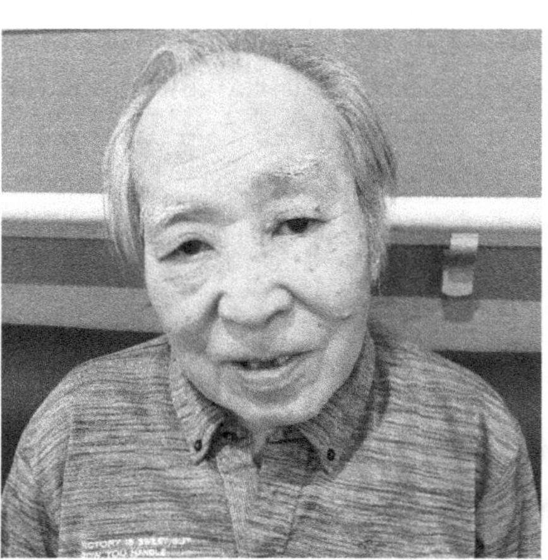

Mr. Nakagawa shows more positive emotions than before.

Urinary or fecal incontinence is a hygiene and privacy issue, and it can also lead to secondary accidents such as causing other residents to slip and fall. Therefore, to help Mr. Nakagawa understand the location of the toilet, we put up a toilet pictogram with the words "toilet here" on the common toilet door and the toilet door in his room. This allowed Mr. Nakagawa to acknowledge the location of toilets and go to the toilet on his own, therefore eliminating urinary and fecal incontinence. To further create a relaxing environment for Mr. Nakagawa, we encouraged him to make use of the sofas installed in the common space. Eventually, he became fond of the sofa at the entrance to the dining room, where he spends time sitting or lying down when he is not eating. He would sometimes sleep on that sofa after going to the toilet at night instead of returning to his room. A place that is comfortable to stay allows him to relax.

Mr. Nakagawa is very fond of his daughter and her husband (son-in-law) and believes one of our caregivers to be his son-in-law. He calls this caregiver by his son-in-law's name and enjoys having conversations whenever this caregiver is assisting him. This caregiver provides care by pretending to be the son-in-law, such as by addressing Mr. Nakagawa the same way the son-in-law would. Incorporating aspects of Lateral Care as such has helped Mr. Nakagawa live in an even more relaxed manner.

According to Mr. Nakagawa's family, he became depressed after losing his wife and almost never left his house. Through our various measures, he has gradually begun to show positive emotions. His family has commented, "his facial expression has become more relaxed. The words he can use have increased as well and we can have more conversations now."

Case 3 Providing Care According to the Current "Reality": Supporting Acceptance

Yaeko Matsui (pseudonym), age 82, devotedly provided care for her husband for 30 years. After her husband passed away, she started showing symptoms of dementia, such as an inability to clean up her home and neglecting her meals, so she moved to Housenka. Mrs. Matsui's dementia was at Stage 4 according to Housenka's dementia progression chart.

After moving in, Mrs. Matsui made a friend, and the two of them enjoyed having coffee at the facility's restaurant and taking walks together. However, when her friend's condition deteriorated and they were no longer able to spend time with each other, Mrs. Matsui became restless, started wandering, and showed increasing signs of anxiety. At this stage, there were three major issues that Mrs. Matsui was experiencing.

The first is that she would often ask, "Where did my husband go?" and search for her dead husband. Now in such cases, we will first show her the photo of her husband that is displayed at the Buddhist altar in her room and try to convey the fact that he has passed away. While she would be able to understand and accept the fact at times, other times, she would insist that it is a stranger's altar and continue to search for her husband. In that case, we acknowledge Mrs. Matsui's "reality" is that her husband is alive but has just gone somewhere and respond as such. For example, if she asks, "Where did my husband go?" we answer, "I wonder where he went too." And if she asks, "Did he go to a higher floor?" we respond, "Let's go look for him together." Oftentimes, when we offer to look for him together, she might say "If he's around, I'm satisfied," and stop searching for him. She may not be able to comprehend the fact that he passed away, but it seems that she knows the truth somewhere in her mind and is trying to sort those emotions in her own way.

The second issue is that sometimes she would be searching for a child. There are two key phrases: one is "Where did that child go?" and the other is "Where did that girl go?" What we learned from the various conversations and Mrs. Matsui's reaction was that the "that child" in the question "Where did that child go?" seems to refer to her grown-up children. When we respond that they are at work, she looks satisfied.

On the other hand, the question "Where did that girl go?" is accompanied by specific statements that seem to be hallucinations or delusions, such as "She just ran past here," or "She was playing here before." It is not clear whether Mrs. Matsui is seeing a "reality" where her children are still young, or a "reality" where there is a park or the like in her view, but when we reply, "I didn't see her," she is somewhat satisfied and does not pursue the matter further. The difference between "that child" and "that girl"" was only discovered after our caregivers discussed their experiences caring for Mrs. Matsui. The fact that Mrs. Matsui would tilt her head in confusion when a caregiver gave the wrong response suggested that there was a clear distinction between the two phrases in her mind.

The third issue was a refusal to bathe. There were concerns since reducing the frequency of bathing is unsanitary, but this issue was quickly solved when Mrs. Matsui made a new friend at Housenka. She gradually started to accompany her friend whenever the friend took a bath, so bathing assistance became smoother with the cooperation of her friend.

As a result of these various measures, Mrs. Matsui began to spend her days peacefully with her new friends, and even began to happily accompany her friend if she was invited to bathe. She also recognized that she has a role, and prepares the residents' cups, tea, and water at mealtime. This was a spontaneous initiative that began when she saw one of our caregivers preparing, and it shows the caring side of Mrs. Matsui, who used to enjoy providing hospitality to house guests.

Assigning roles to a resident is also part of Logical Care. If Mrs. Matsui forgets to prepare the beverages, she will quickly remember her role when a caregiver reminds her. This kind of communication based on fact shows that Logical Care is effective. In addition, since Mrs. Matsui still recognizes the concept of socializing with friends, and since people are often positively influenced by others, it is important for her to continue having good relationships with friends to maintain her quality of life (QOL).

This case is also a typical example of Integrative Care in that Logical Care and Lateral Care are both used according to the situation. Although there are some differences in Mrs. Matsui's reactions, words, and actions depending on the situation, and her mood and calmness fluctuates throughout the day, we will continue to support her by assessing key phrases and the degree of acceptance she expresses.

Case 4 Searching for Reasons From Keywords: Reducing the Desires to Return Home

Chizuko Aida (pseudonym), age 84, was living with her daughter after her husband passed away but entered Housenka when her dementia symptoms advanced. Mrs. Aida's dementia was at Stage 3 according to Housenka's dementia progression chart.

Mrs. Aida was able to conduct personal care, such as dressing, eating, and toileting on her own, and she would even help other residents. She was also able to verbally communicate with us if she had any questions, so Logical Care was applied. However, there was one situation when Logical Care just did not work. This was when she expressed a desire to return home every evening. Normally, Mrs. Aida is able to acknowledge and accept facts, but in this situation, she could not accept the facts no matter how many times the caregivers tried to explain that she now lives in Housenka. She would call her family or the police on her cellphone to complain that she is being confined to the facility, or bang on the door of the staff room until late at night, screaming to let her go home. This issue was very stressful for Mrs. Aida, and it could have led to insomnia or mental and physical problems. As we were searching for solutions, we discovered a clue in the phrases she uses when expressing a desire to return home.

Mrs. Aida would often say something like, "I'm worried about my family, so I want to go home," or "It's getting late, so I want to go home," which is common for those who express desires to return home. However, we also noticed that sometimes, she would say something more specific like, "I'm done with my work, so I want to go home," or "I completed my role, so I want to go home." It seemed that in her mind, there were times when Mrs. Aida had some kind of job or role and wanted to be allowed to return home because she had finished her duties. Her assessment sheet showed that while Mrs. Aida never had a job, according to her family, she was very involved in volunteer activities when she was younger. Therefore, we hypothesized that when Mrs. Aida expresses a desire to return home, in her "reality," she is at the facility to volunteer and wishes to return home once her duties are complete and decided to implement Lateral Care in those situations.

When she would express her desires, instead of trying to make her accept the facts, we would respond as if Mrs. Aida would be going home after she finishes volunteering, such as by saying, "Since we prepared dinner today, why don't you rest here and go home in the morning," or "Your daughter will pick you up, so please wait here for a bit." In some cases, these responses based on Lateral Care satisfied her and helped her calm down. However, in other cases, even if we respond with the same phrase, Mrs. Aida would say, "Why am I leaving?" and "Don't I live here?" In those cases, it means that she has some acknowledgment of the fact that she lives at Housenka and is not visiting for volunteer activities. While the act of expressing a desire to return home is the same, there are times when Mrs. Aida can acknowledge and accept the "fact" that she lives at Housenka, while other times, she is living in a "reality" where she is coming to the facility to volunteer. As we further explored her responses and words, we discovered that the keywords to determining which state she was in were "work," "role" and "volunteer." Although it is not always true, if she mentions "work," "role," or "volunteer," it usually means she is in her "reality" where she is volunteering. On the other hand, if she does not mention those words, there is a high possibility that she will be able to accept "facts."

We decided that we needed to implement Integrative Care and instantly assess Mrs. Aida's state of mind to choose between Logical Care or Lateral Care each time. Although Mrs. Aida continues to express her desire to return home regularly, we quickly respond based on her state of mind. The implementation of Integrative Care has allowed Mrs. Aida and the caregivers to relax a little bit more than before.

Case 5 Completely Affirming the "As Is": From Hell to Paradise

The last case study is about a resident who had been acting bizarrely due to symptoms of dementia, but who regained her composure through Integrative Care.

Kimie Hayashi (pseudonym), age 80, started to show signs of dementia in her late 70's, such as incoherent speech and forgetfulness. She was certified as in-need of nursing care at age 79. Around this time, her bizarre behavior escalated, perhaps due to the progression of cognitive symptoms. She would sleep in the common hallways of her apartment, leave soiled underwear due to incontinence all over her room, rush into police or fire stations late at night, and stay at the city office all day to complain about what seemed like delusions, such as someone breaking into her house to destroy her toilet.

Complaints were received from various places, and the family was at a complete loss of what to do. Mrs. Hayashi was using an elder day care service, but she was unable to adjust to the environment, and there was no place that would accept her for short-stay programs. That was the situation when Mrs. Hayashi's family contacted Housenka to ask for help.

The family wanted Mrs. Hayashi to move into a Housenka facility that was close to her home, but at the time, it was still under construction and would not open for another two months. However, the family was at their limit, and could not continue to care for Mrs. Hayashi during that time. It was decided that she would be accepted at a Housenka facility in another area for a short-stay program and move into the new facility when it opened. Even though we knew that this decision had risks, she entered Housenka at age 79. Mrs. Hayashi's dementia was at Stage 5 according to Housenka's dementia progression chart. The dementia has since been diagnosed as Alzheimer's disease.

The first issue was that she was not receiving appropriate support and medical care for her cognitive symptoms because she would strongly refuse any treatment. Care managers and the community comprehensive support center advised us that Mrs. Hayashi should be transferred to a psychiatric hospital. However, we knew that there was a possibility that her vitality would decline due to physical restraints and medication that would be inevitable if she were sent to a psychiatric hospital in this condition. We politely declined the advice and accepted her, while searching for a different option where we could provide appropriate care that would allow her to live at Housenka comfortably.

Before Mrs. Hayashi moved in, we conducted an interview with her. When we asked her if she went to the city office almost every day, she replied, "Yes, I will make a complaint," signaling that she recognizes the facts. However, when we asked her the reason and content of the complaint, she could not give a coherent answer. She would clearly express that she disliked all kinds of elder care facilities, including Housenka, by continuing to angrily shout, "I won't enter a place like this, I'm going home" in an agitated state.

It was winter, so letting her out of the facility would strain her body. It was also true that her toilet in her home was broken. When we said,

"Since your toilet is broken and it would be dangerous if you get into trouble with various people again, why not spend some time here to calm down?" she continued to yell but reluctantly accepted the use of our short-stay program. We decided that Logical Care was appropriate since she could still have coherent conversations to some degree.

Once she moved in, she continued to yell at us every time we tried to care for her. After some time, she finally began to show minor signs of being relaxed. We decided it was time to move to the next step—bathing care—while cautiously making sure we did not overstep any boundaries. Her family told us that Mrs. Hayashi had not bathed for about two years. A short time after she moved in, she started accepting full-body wiping, but she continued to stubbornly refuse to bathe. Mrs. Hayashi insisted that she could not bathe because she had pneumonia, but she did not show any symptoms and a physician also confirmed that she did not have pneumonia.

Then one day, Mrs. Hayashi complained of her feet itching. We saw this as an opportunity, and nervously suggested a foot bath. To our surprise, not only did she accept, but she also fell in love with foot baths. We did not want to miss this chance, so after helping her take foot baths in her room for several weeks, we changed the location to the bathroom. Once she was adjusted to the new environment, we monitored her mood, and suggested washing her hair when she was in a good mood. She also accepted this suggestion, and after many sessions of washing her hair, she finally accepted a full shower. Although she did not recover to the point of taking a bath, this was the outcome of assigning a dedicated caregiver to thoroughly care for Mrs. Hayashi to build a trusting relationship with her.

Around the time that she came to accept showers and finally began to lead a more relaxed life, the new facility near her home opened. We informed the family that staying in the current facility was also an option, but they requested a transfer to the new facility. After she moved, the risks that we feared were realized. The new environment caused Mrs. Hayashi to become very confused and furiously yelled, "Where the hell am I?", "Why the hell did you bring me to this damned place?", and "I don't trust you people." On the day she moved in, she caused so much commotion that the other residents looked at her, puzzled, to see what was going on, while our caregivers looked on from a distance; this created a bizarre atmosphere.

She continued to be suspicious of others, such as carrying all of her belongings with her, and sitting on a chair in the facility restaurant and covering herself with a blanket to sleep instead of in her own room. Our caregivers patiently accompanied Mrs. Hayashi in pairs without denying anything she said or did and continued to care for her by affirming her in every way. The actions of our caregivers finally loosened her up. About two weeks later, she was able to understand her situation better and accepted that the facility was a safe place with no enemies. She started to act in a more relaxed manner.

We felt that Mrs. Hayashi tended to accept the situation better if caregivers acknowledged her thoughts and accommodate her wishes, so we decided to continue this method. After one month, she began to lean against the wall to sleep sitting on her own bed, and after another month, she began to sleep lying down on the bed, eventually reaching a point where she is now sleeping comfortably on her bed. She also started leaving her belongings in her own room. Furthermore, there were more occasions when she could have coherent conversations and her memory also seemed to improve.

Since she had a better grasp of her current location, she was also able to return safely to the facility as long as her destination was a certain distance from the facility. In a little over a month, her relationship with our caregivers also changed dramatically. At first, the caregivers would walk a step behind Mrs. Hayashi while she would express her displeasure about the situation. Eventually, she would not show displeasure even if a caregiver walked next to her to talk, and finally, she was able to safely walk on her own while caregivers gently watched her from behind. One time, she tripped and fell and broke her left cheekbone. While this was an unfortunate accident, there was also a silver lining. Mrs. Hayashi had a CT scan taken when she went to the hospital, which officially diagnosed her dementia. We believe that she was able to acknowledge her condition and accept the need for treatment as an outcome of Logical Care.

As we stated earlier, Mrs. Hayashi was able to take a shower for the first time in two years while she was using Housenka's short-stay program. However, we had to start from scratch when she transferred to the new facility since she returned to a state where she refused bathing because she insisted that she had pneumonia. We had a physician explain that the pneumonia had been cured but she would still not be satisfied. After some discussion we decided to implement Lateral Care and tune into her "reality" where she has pneumonia. Then, little by little, changes began to appear. First, we were able to perform full-body wiping according to her complaints of itchiness. After more time had passed, she resumed accepting foot baths. When she complained that her hair was uncomfortable, she would accept washing her hair at the hair salon within the facility. As we continued to accommodate her desires in this way, she started accepting more things, and eventually returned to accepting showers. However, she again started refusing showers when winter arrived, so we performed full-body wiping while looking for an opportunity where she would accept showering or bathing.

When I heard the report that Mrs. Hayashi had started accepting showers again, I was very proud of our caregivers at Housenka, who treat the residents with sincerity and dedication. This was a very difficult case since Mrs. Hayashi's memories and mindset constantly shifted between past and present as well as reality and unreality. However, this is the type of situation where Integrative Care really shows its value.

These days, Mrs. Hayashi is leading a comfortable and relaxed life. As she has become calmer, her relationship with her family and other residents has improved. At first, her family avoided visiting Mrs. Hayashi for fear of her constant yelling and screaming, but now they are very happy that they can visit regularly and can occasionally take her out of the facility.

It is hard to believe that she was isolated and did not interact with anyone at her previous elder day care service. Now, she enjoys talking with everyone, participating in recreational activities, and taking pictures. She has made friends, and in some cases, she even comforts people who are sad. Sometimes she would even say words of encouragement to our caregivers, which shows that she was naturally a very kind person.

Looking at how she behaves these days, I cannot help but wonder if her violent and unruly behavior—which was enough for physicians to suggest hospitalization in a psychiatric hospital—was a reaction to her hellish situation in which she constantly felt like she was being disrespected and treated as a nuisance. Unfortunately, in society, people with dementia are often quickly dismissed due to the prejudice that they will not be able to understand anything anyway. However, I believe that people with dementia can sense that they are being viewed this way. This may be why Mrs. Hayashi was acting bizarrely; it was actually a desperate effort to announce her existence.

At Housenka, we respond to residents head-on and explain everything carefully and thoroughly. The sincerity of our efforts must have reached Mrs. Hayashi, who may be thinking, "The people here are different from others I met in the past," and "These people follow me for some reason, but they are kind to me," and I believe that this has led to her current condition.

People with dementia who are verbally abusive or violent tend to be labeled as "troubled" people. Even some care managers and other professionals tend to view them as such. As a result, the person with dementia is given an inaccurate diagnosis and driven towards inefficient treatment. It is very unfortunate, but such cases are actually not uncommon.

This case taught us once again the danger of looking at people with dementia through biased views. It is also a great representation of the cardinal rule of care, which is to try everything we can even if other professionals make decisions that seem to be abandoning that person. I believe that properly facing and examining the situation with our own eyes brought about significant progress in this case, and Mrs. Hayashi responded to our efforts.

Now, Mrs. Hayashi has so much vitality, as if she made a huge leap to get from hell to paradise. Although cases with such a remarkable change may be rare, we would like readers to know that such cases actually exist.

The Key to Maintaining Composure: Clearly Define the Pillar of Care

Providing care is not all about accomplishment. Caregivers are often faced with grim situations that are full of raw emotions such as in the cases in this book. Some caregivers may find these situations heartbreaking.

In Mrs. Hayashi's case, our caregivers were able to maintain their composure due to three factors: (1) their professionalism, (2) the fact that several staff members were able to take turns providing care, and (3) the fact that they could sense even the slightest changes in Mrs. Hayashi.

Eyes that detect changes can also be considered a meticulous eye for observation, which is indispensable for Integrative Care.

"Professionalism" means to clearly understand the mission as caregivers and clarify the desired outcomes. During Housenka's training sessions, we teach our new caregivers that our purpose as caregivers is to solve problems in society and to bring about positive change for our residents, and that we must always ask ourselves what is necessary to achieve this and share our ideas. We believe that as long as the care being provided has a clearly defined pillar, we can maintain an objective perspective to fulfill our purpose, even when we are treated harshly by residents or their families. By practicing care with this mentality and experiencing success, we are able to expect further positive changes in our residents. In other words, we can find enjoyment and pleasure in care.

Having said that, replicating professionalism and taking turns with care may be difficult if when taking care of a person with dementia at home. As a result, caregivers may not even have the luxury to perceive any changes (as stated in item 3). If you feel that you cannot handle the situation on your own or at a loss of what to do, do not think that you have to be responsible for everything. Make sure to seek help from outside parties or professionals. In particular, it is best to avoid an environment where the person with dementia is not accepted or is disrespected by those around them. Focus on finding a facility that allows that person to be who they are as much as possible and professionals who believe in that kind of care.

On the other hand, we would also like to state that care at a professional facility is not the only option. It is also quite possible for families to provide efficient care at home based on the methods introduced in this book. Participants of the Green Oasis Meeting—a family meeting hosted by Housenka (see "Introduction")—have commented that they are now able to affirm the actions of the person with dementia, or that their strained relationships have improved after accepting their actions and words. The words and actions of a person with dementia are difficult to understand from the perspective of the general public, therefore it is difficult to fully affirm them. However, this affirmation is the key to dementia care. We encourage you to practice truly affectionate care by first removing your own mental models.

Chapter 6
A New Age of Dementia Care

People with Dementia Can Still Perform ADL!

Despite Resident's Brain Atrophy, the Results Surprise Even Physicians

In previous chapters, we explored our three new methods of dementia care: Logical Care (Fact Acceptance-Based Aid), Lateral Care (Reality Affirmation-Based Aid), and Integrative Care (Comprehensive Aid).

When we presented the prototypes of these methods at the Housenka Group's research and development (R&D) presentation in the summer of 2015, we received a great deal of criticism. Some of the comments we received were, "I don't understand what you're trying to say," "Allowing a resident to sleep on the couch is outrageous," and "Why can't we give the residents chopsticks or spoons?" These reactions reminded us of how caregivers (including me) have been bound by our own mental models of "common sense" and "ideals," and have been imposing them on people with dementia.

While the methods have received numerous criticisms, I am confident that these methods are effective. This confidence is based on a single important factor: the facial expressions of the residents. It is a fact that our residents' facial expressions changed dramatically after we began practicing the three new methods. Those who used to have worried, grim, or angry expressions on their faces now have lively, relaxed expressions on their faces; some even show us their sweetest smiles. It has also alleviated the residents' restlessness and decreased how frequently they refuse care. Many of them eat and sleep better now, allowing them to lead a more peaceful life.

A family member of one resident who has been diagnosed with Alzheimer's disease almost 15 years ago said, "My mother's progression is definitely slower than that of someone I know with Alzheimer's disease who lives in another facility. The difference may be in the care they receive." This is an example that shows that the care provided affects the deterioration speed and the ability to complete activities of daily living (ADL), and that our new methods are effective.

A physician who saw a CT image of one of our resident's brains has told us, "I am amazed at the resident's ability to complete ADL even with all this brain atrophy." There are many such cases where the medical evidence does not correlate with the actual ability to complete ADL. Of course, it is important for those with severe symptoms to take prescribed medications, but not all people who take medications are able to maintain their ability to complete ADL.

To reiterate, the goal of our dementia care is to bring out the "will to live" in each resident by affirming and respecting all aspects of their lives. In other words, it is an effort to support the will to live. **We believe that true dementia care should not focus on maintaining cognitive functions, but rather on maintaining the ability to complete ADL, which is directly linked to the will to live.** The ability to maintain this ability depends on the type of care provided by caregivers.

Support That Allows Maximum Independent Living

What should family members keep in mind for the person with dementia to retain their ability to complete ADL? This is a topic that comes up in the Green Oasis Meeting, a family meeting hosted by Housenka, since it is a common concern.

The families often comment on how they end up doing everything for the person with dementia for reasons such as not knowing what the person is still able to do and not having the time or leisure to wait for the person to do it on their own. Doing everything for the person certainly takes less time and is easier for both the person and the caregiver. However, continuing to do so will cause the abilities of people with dementia to quickly deteriorate and eventually completely disappear. The other extreme, also common when families that care for people with dementia at home, are attempts by families to try to force a person to learn or complete ADL as much as possible regardless of that person's remaining abilities. This can lead to the person being forced to do something that their abilities no longer allow them to do or situations where that person is disrespected for not being able to do a certain task, which in turn leads to the person becoming demoralized or discouraged. The important thing is to not dismiss the person's behavior and encourage their acceptance of the situation so that they are able to complete ADL to the best of their abilities. This is the secret to maintaining the abilities to complete ADL.

Even those who are considered by their families to be incapable of functioning in daily life learn to be able to do many things once they move into Housenka. Actually, it is arrogant for us to say we "taught" them how to function; they probably already had the ability to do these things in the first place. Singing cheerfully, eating without assistance, conversing with others, making tea for everyone; these are some of the activities that surprise families when they come to visit. They may say, "I can't believe grandma learned how to do this," but we believe that it just means that she already knew how but did not have the opportunity to use her abilities while she was being cared for at home.

The essence of dementia care is to determine what an individual can do in certain aspects of their daily life, and to provide care that allows them to live independently as much as possible. To put it simply, we must assess their remaining abilities and allow them to use them as much as possible. If it is an ability that allows them to perform activities that would be of assistance to others, the person may become more motivated and regain even more abilities, to the surprise of family members and even professional caregivers.

In addition, regular health checkups are essential to maintain abilities to complete ADL. People with dementia may not notice changes in their own physical condition even if they develop another disease, or if they do notice, they may not be able to express their condition well enough. As a result, that disease may progress unnoticed, which can be fatal. Dental checkups and oral care are also important. Cavities, missing teeth, ill-fitting dentures, malocclusion, or the like can lead to oral problems, which can interfere with food intake, cause mouth sores and pain, and induce disease due to discomfort or poor hygiene.

To eliminate such situations as much as possible, we would like to encourage our readers to discard stereotypes and assumptions, such as "People with dementia will be reluctant or unable to undergo checkups," "They are elderly and no longer need checkups," or "They are fine because they see a physician regularly." Instead, have the person with dementia undergo regular health checkups. Checkups are also useful as an objective assessment of that person's health.

Health is an Ability: The Concept of Positive Health

Leading a Meaningful Life Even With Dementia

Even if one has dementia, wanting to maintain abilities to complete ADL and live a healthy life is very important. This idea is similar to the concept of "positive health," which was proposed in the Netherlands in 2011 and is currently attracting attention around the world. Dr. Machteld Huber, a Dutch family physician and proponent of the concept, defines health as "people's ability to deal with physical, emotional and social challenges in life—and to be in charge of their own affairs, whenever possible." She claims that health cannot be defined as "a state without illness or disability," in today's society, and that the new concept of health should be to live positively even with an illness or disability by utilizing the people and things around on one's own initiative.

Objective Health and Subjective Health

I strongly agree with Dr. Huber. Up until now, health was seen as a "state." The common perception was that health is a state in which one has no physical, mental, or social problems—or in other words, a state without illness or disability. However, such a state is often not possible in today's society. The reality is that almost everyone is living with some kind of illness or disability. Instead of focusing on a "state" based on having a disease or disability, such a society should emphasize how that person can achieve a better life. This "ability" to achieve a better life is the core concept of positive health.

Based on this idea, even if a person has dementia, they should be able to live comfortably and enhance their own life by using a variety of resources. According to the original concept of positive health, this must be achieved through self-management, but this is often difficult for people with dementia. However, people with dementia also have opinions, wishes and urges. Therefore, family members or we, as professional caregivers, provide care based on assessments.

I believe that there are two sides to health that are equally important: objective health and subjective health. The former refers to the presence of illness or disability, treatment of physical, emotional, and social problems, and determination of health conditions based on numerical values and other objective data obtained from regular health checkups. The latter is comparable to positive health and refers to the ability to lead a meaningful and satisfying life even with dementia or another illness by making use of various social resources and alternative functions. In other words, I believe that the environment around a person—the people around, resources available, etc. —greatly influences that person's quality of life (QOL).

Many people believe that they must give up a comfortable life, social contact, and sense of purpose because of their illness. Those diagnosed with dementia, in particular, often suffer tremendous anxiety when they think about the loss of memory, judgment, and comprehension that is associated with dementia. However, it is possible to maintain subjective health and abilities to complete ADL, or more specifically, to pursue moments of happiness, if the loss of abilities caused by dementia can be compensated for with some assistance. I believe that such a society can be realized, depending on how dementia care evolves.

Just in Case: Prepare a "Dementia Notebook"

In addition to creating an environment that supports a person with dementia, it is also important for the person themselves to prepare if they wish to lead a fulfilling life as before. For example, in recent years, an increasing number of people have been preparing an end-of-life planning notebook as part of their end-of-life planning activities, and I think it would be a good idea to prepare a dementia notebook to prepare for the onset of dementia in the same way.

As seen in the case studies, the behavior of a person with dementia is often linked to their past. Even though there is a possibility that your preferences and particularities may change with the onset of dementia, it is important to have a summary of one's life and medical history, the desired lifestyle and care style (home or facility, etc.), personal preferences, and wishes at the time of death, in case verbal communication becomes difficult. This will be a useful tool that will help caregivers to understand when the time comes. The existence of such a notebook will also make it easier for one's family to provide care. If possible, discuss with professionals what social resources are available. It is important to express our wishes while we can still communicate, especially if we are elderly and at a higher risk of developing dementia.

In Japan, death and money tend to be taboo subjects, but we have seen many families who, once a family member develops dementia and are unable to communicate, find themselves in chaos because they do not know where that person's bank books are, what assets they have, or what kind of end-of-life care they desire. If an individual does not have family or someone else they trust, they may want to use the adult conservatorship system. We recommend that people prepare in advance before they or their family members develop dementia.

You Are the One Who Best Understands the Person With Dementia

Learning From the Person With Dementia

Through our care studies of Logical Care, Lateral Care, and Integrative Care, we have explained how the environment surrounding a person with dementia can change their daily life or even their whole life.

There are many things in that environment that caregivers can influence. It is clear that the relationship between the person with dementia and the caregiver is extremely important. This is true for both family members and professional caregivers. *You* the caregiver are the best person to understand the person before you who is seeking help.

As the people with the greatest understanding, we should not only support those with dementia, but also be willing to learn from them. Here, I would like to appeal to care professionals in particular. At Housenka, residents with various symptoms teach us many things. In fact, we were only able to develop our new methods because our residents have given us many insights.

Learning from the person with dementia and asking them to teach us what we lack will lead to respect for that person. When caregivers treat people with respect and warmth, it directly leads to the enrichment of the lives of those people. No matter how good the physical environment is, if the family members or caregivers who are supposed to be providing support and assistance lack the perspective of "maintaining the ability to complete ADL," "providing care that draws out the power to live," and "enhancing vitality and life," that good environment will be completely meaningless.

While the physical aspects of support are important in care, the human aspect of support is even more important. And it is the mindset of the caregiver that determines the quality of that human aspect. For a person with dementia, the caregiver who supports them with sincerity is a big part of their lives. I believe that this is a fact that all caregivers really need to take to heart.

Failures are Inevitable: Make the Most of Them in Your Next Step

It is also undeniable that many caregivers involved in dementia care experience burnout syndrome due to the heavy responsibilities and workload. Communication with a person with dementia can be difficult, and the person may refuse your care. At times, they may even yell at or hit you. You may feel that your passion to support the person with dementia is not enough and have doubts about continuing. How one views these experiences, for a professional caregiver is the fork in your career path.

"Failure," as we might label these experiences, is not a bad thing; it is a necessary process in order to achieve the desired outcomes. For example, although I have published books in which I describe dementia care methods and various case studies, I still experience failure at times when I actually work in the field. There is no such thing as dementia care without failures. That is why it is important to use your experiences of failure to improve your own skills.

All experiences, including failures, can help us cultivate experiential knowledge such as "I should provide this type of care in such situations," and "This method didn't work so I'll try another one." By cultivating this knowledge, applying dementia care methods in practice from various perspectives, and theorizing based on the actual events taking place in the field, we will be able to see new things. This is what learning from practice means. We must be careful not to let our practice be dictated solely by the methods we introduced or our theories.

In the case studies introduced in this book, we have not been shy about sharing our trial-and-error experiences. In many cases, we tested method A first, switched to method B when A did not work, then to C if B did not work, and so on. By learning from practice—in other words, being taught by residents—repeatedly, we were able to shift from "just having knowledge" to "using that knowledge to handle a situation."

I sincerely hope that caregivers involved in dementia care will not despair at their first failure and will have the resilience to base innovations on these failures.

The Ten Principles of Dementia Care

What must one keep in mind when practicing dementia care? Here are ten principles to remember when practicing our new methods.

(1) Acquire Information for Successful Communication.

Start by getting to know the person with dementia. If you are a professional caregiver, acquire information by gaining the understanding and cooperation of family members. You can increase your rate of successful communication with the person with dementia if you are able to discover keywords as you gain information from the family, instead of just drawing on superficial information. Remember to also doubt your own mental model to some degree.

(2) Understand the Person's Feelings and Behavior.

If the person clearly expresses their needs, the problem can be solved by listening to the person carefully and providing support in accordance with their complaints. However, in some cases, the person may not be able to express their true needs. Therefore, it is crucial to be able to detect the person's true needs through changes in facial expressions, behavior, and the like. It is especially important to look at their eyes to gain information.

(3) Use Visualization and Other Communication Methods.

People with dementia may not be able to understand verbal communication, but they may be able to understand visually. For example, even if they do not understand the words "wash your hands," they may be able to wash their hands on their own if they see a sink. Rather than giving up on communicating just because the person does not understand your words, try to use other methods that the person can understand, such as visual communication.

(4) Do Not Stop Them Immediately.

Unless it is dangerous or a nuisance to others, try not to stop the person's behavior immediately. Consider the behavior as information. This new information, combined with other information, may lead to a new awareness that will lead to better care.

(5) Do Not Dismiss Any Behavior.

If you try to discover the significance behind the person's behavior instead of dismissing it, you may understand the meaning of that behavior.

(6) Respond According to the Person's Ability, Condition and Situation.

dementia care must be provided according to the person's abilities, condition, and situation. Decide whether to provide Logical Care, Lateral Care, or Integrative Care by observing whether communication is being established successfully, whether you are channeled into the correct "reality," etc.

(7) White Lies are Necessary at Times.

The outcomes of dementia care depend on whether the person with dementia is satisfied with the situation. Sometimes it is necessary to lie or reframe the facts for the person to be satisfied and relaxed.

(8) Do Not Put Stress on the Person.

Stress will definitely aggravate the person's condition. There are many things that can cause stress, such as providing care based on your "normal" and "ideals," so refrain from such activities.

(9) Know the Person's "Reality."

To provide efficient care, you must channel into their current "reality." Providing care based on the wrong "reality" will be inefficient and will only cause stress for both of you. In dementia care, it is essential that you act to suit the person's convenience, rather than trying to make the person suit our "normal" convenience. If the person becomes distressed, it is important to make sure you are acting for their needs, while channeled into their "reality."

(10) Match Words and Actions.

The foundation of dementia care is to be consistent in what you say and do when providing care. A person without dementia can complain about inconsistencies in our words and actions, but a person with dementia cannot, leading only to stress. The caregiver must always be mindful of matching their words and actions.

Just following these principles is not enough to practice Logical Care, Lateral Care, and Integrative Care. As we communicate with the person, we must determine which of the three methods is appropriate and find the support that the person truly needs. We have repeatedly stated that there is no universal solution for dementia care. Dementia care cannot be provided solely based on knowledge. The essence of dementia care is to use the knowledge acquired and patiently attempt communication repeatedly, which may be difficult at times, in order to organize the situation on the spot and provide appropriate care.

If you are a professional caregiver, we would like you to keep these ten principles in mind, and perseveringly gain experience through practice. There is no need to aim for a perfect score at every moment.

The Two Paradigm Shifts to Realize Better Care

The ten principles described above are only techniques and means, and to provide better care, we must always keep in mind the desired outcome, which are the purpose and goals of the care. The ten principles are merely concepts that serve to achieve the desired outcome. The desired outcome, needless to say, is to bring happiness and comfort to the life of the person with dementia. Throughout this book, we have presented the following two paradigm shifts that must occur to achieve this outcome. The first is Logical Care, Lateral Care, and Integrative Care, which in short, are communication techniques.

Logical Care should be applied first in most cases, but as we better understand the person with dementia, we can switch to Lateral Care or Integrative Care to help the person accept and become satisfied with the situation. It is important to have an eye to quickly determine which care is the most effective.

The other paradigm shift that must occur is to become aware of our mental models. This means recognizing that our own thoughts and actions are based on our mental models. As mentioned earlier, a mental model is the subconscious mind of an individual that guides their thoughts, and includes assumptions, values, and common sense. The subconscious mind is formed throughout past experiences. In other words, past experiences form mental models, which form the basis for our thoughts, which in turn guides our words and actions. As we stated in Chapter 2, stereotyping, unconscious bias, and paternalism make up a good portion of our mental model.

Change Your Mindset to Break Free From Mental Models

Stereotypes are preconceptions based on assumptions and fixed views. Examples include "One must eat three meals a day," "Food must be eaten with utensils," or "People should only sleep on beds or futons."

Unconscious bias is an unconscious evaluation of a person, action, situation, or the like. While it is an important function in making quick judgments, it may also prevent us from making conscious judgments. For example, quickly deciding, "The person has dementia, so I will explain it in an easy-to-understand way" is an unconscious bias. On the other hand, thinking "The person has dementia so they cannot understand or do anything," is also an unconscious bias. When unconscious bias works in the wrong direction, it can lead to negative judgments, such as "Eating with your hands is embarrassing, dirty, and can lead to burns," "Sleeping on a sofa is not good for your health," "The person has dementia so they are incoherent, and I can dismiss them," or "Elders do not have to put on makeup." Care based on these judgements will not be efficient.

Paternalism occurs when a professional or authority figure unilaterally supports a person (especially a vulnerable person) based on that professional's or authority figure's own values, without listening carefully to another person's wishes or story, because they believe it is in the best interest of the other person. This is a phenomenon brought about by caregivers' intentions to ensure that the person with dementia is not disadvantaged due to the cognitive impairments that do not allow them to make proper decisions. An example of paternalism would be a caregiver who believes that serving three well-balanced and calorie-calculated meals a day is the key to health and who continues to serve the same meals without considering the individual's dietary patterns and preferences.

Other examples include thinking that we are not fulfilling our duties if the person with dementia is not on a regular schedule, or conducting actions out of fear that others will think that we are not providing proper care, such as bathing them on a regular schedule regardless of their desires, not allowing them to leave their seats during mealtimes even if they remember something they must do, or restraining them or limiting their rights so they do not fall and break a bone while wandering.

While stereotypes, unconscious bias, and paternalism might serve a purpose, we must understand that these can obstruct appropriate dementia care. As we mentioned in Chapter 2, if we do not acknowledge them, the care we provide might not take the person's expressions or the like into account or be solely based on common care theories. To change this behavior, we must first change our mindsets. We must recognize that people with dementia live in their own unique worlds and cultures and acknowledge their diversity. This is one of the most important aspects of dementia care.

Similarities With Diversity and Inclusion

Unconscious bias, assumptions, and the like that have a negative impact on communication are seen not only in dementia care, but also in many other aspects of modern society.

Today, as globalization advances, the world is working to create a society in which people of diverse races and cultures can live in harmony with each other. You may have heard the term "diversity and inclusion," which emphasizes generosity towards all. At the same time, there is also a focus on unconscious bias, which is an obstacle to diversity and inclusion. Corporate training to help employees become aware of the existence of unconscious bias is being conducted in various companies around the world, including Google and Starbucks.

Some of you may not see the similarities in dementia care with the mindset necessary to respect each other in a multilingual, multicultural, and multiracial environment. In the case of global interactions, both parties must mutually devote efforts to understand and respect each other. On the other hand, in dementia care, the relationship between the two parties may not be equal since it requires a strong compromise on the part of the caregivers. However, the caregiver must think about how to accept the current "reality" of the person with dementia, and respect and understand the difficult world the person lives in. To this end, they must be aware of their own stereotypes, unconscious bias, and paternalism, and be able to consciously form other appropriate responses.

I believe that this new mindset, which is important for successful communication, is common to both diversity and inclusion and dementia care. Stereotypes, unconscious bias, and paternalism sometimes lead us to behaviors that offend the dignity of others and disrespect their values. We must be aware of this fact and constantly remind ourselves of it.

Taking steps toward small realizations will gradually cause your actions to change, which will also change the results of your care. If the results change and you are exposed to successful outcomes such as maintaining the potential and ability of the person to complete ADL, or their relaxed or happy expressions, your mental model will change, which will also lead to your thoughts, actions, and words to change. All this in turn leads to the expansion of possibilities and the creation of a peaceful life for those with dementia. In other words, a positive spiral of dementia care is created.

To Realize a Dementia Care Paradise

Nonverbal Communication Through Technology

Our definition of "dementia care paradise" is a place where people with dementia can enjoy as much freedom as possible, where their dignity is protected and their existence, words, and actions are respected.

Assumptions and impositions, such as assuming that the person with dementia will not be able to understand or imposing socially-acceptable behavior, will cause the person to feel that their dignity was denied. A place where people can be free from such suffering and live as they are without being judged—this is the type of place we wish to realize. Whether or not this paradise has been realized can only be inferred from the facial expressions, words, and actions of those with dementia. However, this judgment is currently left to the subjective judgment of caregivers. While you may think it is easy to tell if a person with dementia is smiling or relaxed, this is also a *subjective* judgment. There is always the possibility that different caregivers will have different standards for judgment.

This is where technology comes into play. The use of technology is expected to increase in the long-term care field, which will give us an objective evaluation. Various research is being conducted to explore the possibility of artificial intelligence (AI) and "the internet of things" (IoT) in nonverbal communication. For example, a patch-type EEG (electroencephalograph), developed by Professor Tsuyoshi Sekitani of Osaka University, can visualize brain conditions easily and in real time, simply by placing a sheet-type wireless EEG sensor on the forehead. Currently, it can also diagnose the types of dementia about 70 to 80 percent of the time, and if this becomes widely used, simple dementia diagnosis can be conducted at nursing homes, local clinics, and homes.

As research progresses and technology advances, it may become possible to understand what a person with dementia is feeling and thinking to some extent by measuring brain waves. Such objective evaluation would make it easier to provide evidence-based care. The realization of nonverbal communication through technology is highly anticipated, as it will be useful not only in the field of dementia care, but also in autism care, palliative care, and other settings.

Medical care and digital devices are advancing rapidly. In the long-term care field, various technologies to assist daily living and activities—so-called assistive technology—are being introduced on a trial basis, in an effort to improve the QOL of those in need. This kind of science-based care is attracting attention as a new option that will be common in the future.

Dementia Care is Not Just a Science

It is common sense to provide evidence-based treatment in the medical field. In recent years, the provision of scientific-evidence based care has also been promoted in the long-term care field. The idea is that providing care that is backed by scientific evidence instead of care that relies only on experience and intuition will contribute to building a sustainable care system in preparation for the growing demand for long-term care.

To expand the use of evidence-based care, vast amounts of data must be collected and analyzed. Physical care in particular, requires scientific evidence to guarantee the quality of care and outcomes, and the professionalism of caregivers who provide non-evidence-based physical therapy will be questioned. On the other hand, unlike physical care, our concept of dementia care—the new methods proposed in this book—

is not based on such scientific data. This is because—as we stated many times before—the symptoms of dementia differ from person to person, even if the type of dementia is the same. In particular, behavioral symptoms are unique to each person since they depend on the person's life history, which includes their personal thoughts, cultures, values, customs, habits, and obsessions, as well as the person's current physical functions.

For example, people tend to think of wandering as a single symptom. However, the reasons (in other words the history of the person) that leads to wandering are different for each individual. If the desired outcome is to completely stop wandering, then having the person take medication that suppresses the behavior may be considered effective. But we must first think about whether or not we should stop wandering in the first place. Care for wandering should be to determine the reason for wandering and provide support based on that reason. There are many possible ways to approach this depending on the reason, and there is not enough evidence to declare that one method is absolutely correct.

While it is important to base dementia care on science, it is also natural that personalized care is required if we consider that the words and actions of those with dementia are based on individual circumstances and situations. For this reason, we feel that it is impossible to explain all aspects of dementia care based on science.

Artistic Creativity Is Required in Dementia Care

Dementia care can be thought of as a fusion of science and art. In addition to understanding the scientific evidence, we believe that dementia care requires the ability to devise ways to connect and communicate with the person, to understand their will and create an environment beneficial to their life. In other words, it requires an artistic talent to "make the invisible visible." Art includes the abilities to perceive a situation and to tactfully respond to that situation, and such abilities are essential for dementia care. In addition, dementia care also requires the ability to see things from the other person's perspective, in other words, to be altruistic, in order to change our role and psychological distance from that person according to the situation. These are very important and indispensable abilities in dementia care, which requires caregivers to "create care based on the present moment."

As seen in the case studies in this book, the detail of care is unique to each individual. In a field where caregivers must constantly think about how to make a person's current condition as comfortable as possible through a combination of care methods and information about that person's life history, symptoms, and the like, it is natural that artistic creativity is required.

In summary, dementia care occurs when the person with dementia and all those who are involved with them work together to shape the life of the person with dementia.

Protect Lives, Enjoy Daily Life, and Enrich Life

The idea that "medicine is both a science and an art" has been proposed in some medical institutions in the United States and elsewhere, but it has not spread to the public yet. This is true especially in Japan, where some people think of science as a higher discipline than art. However, they are equal in value, and both have contributed to the development of human society and culture.

To deal with the complex and personal nature of dementia, it is necessary to integrate the seemingly opposite specialties of art and science at a high level and to view the person with dementia in a comprehensive manner. Instead of drawing a border, the medical field should be actively conscious of the artistic aspect, while the long-term care field should be more conscious of the scientific aspect. We believe this will lead to better collaboration between the two fields.

Ultimately, the capacity to provide integrated nursing and medical care should pave the way to a dementia care paradise.

What can we do now to realize care that allows people with dementia to live independent and peaceful lives without stress and pain in any situation, and that also reduces stress for caregivers? How can we create an environment for people with dementia that protects their lives, lets them enjoy daily life, and enriches their lives? Dementia care that can bring happiness to both the person with dementia and the caregivers starts with seriously considering these issues.

CONCLUSION

Tamae Yamamoto (pseudonym), who started us on the path to our new care methods, is now sadly bedridden most of the time. Scenes of her eating with her hands are now a thing of the past. However, she has not lost her appetite. When we try to feed her with a spoon, she opens her mouth willingly, chews well, and also has no problem swallowing. We are not certain if she still understands our words, but she often nods and relaxes her expressions when we speak to her. Even though she cannot use chopsticks and spoons and can no longer eat with her hands, she has never forgotten the act of eating. And although she cannot communicate verbally, her mind seems to be at ease knowing that she is part of a social circle. Her peaceful life seems to be filled with the joy of living based on her will to live.

She is showing us the spark of her pure vitality, which has been freed from the norms and ties imposed by society as a result of dementia. It is a sight we must pay respect to, and it also gives us vitality and energy. This mutual resonance is perhaps the best part of dementia care.

I would like to conclude this book with a message to family members and professional caregivers who are caring for a person with dementia

First of all, to family members: as I have said throughout, please do not take on the responsibility of caregiving alone or with only your own family members. While there have been many cases of family members providing excellent care that is only possible for them, if the burden is too great, you will not be able to provide it for a long time. It will lead to stress for you, your family, and the person with dementia, which will further trap you in a downward spiral.

In some of the case studies in this book, I feel that we were only able to intervene after the limits of family care had been exceeded. It is important to seek help from professionals before you reach your limit, become discouraged or hopeless. You must speak up to let others know what is troubling you.

When working with specialists, it is important to cooperate with them. There are many things that only family members know, such as the person's personality, lifestyle, and life history. This information is crucial to provide better care. Please understand that effective dementia care is only possible when the person with dementia, the family, and the professionals work together to shape the person's environment and life.

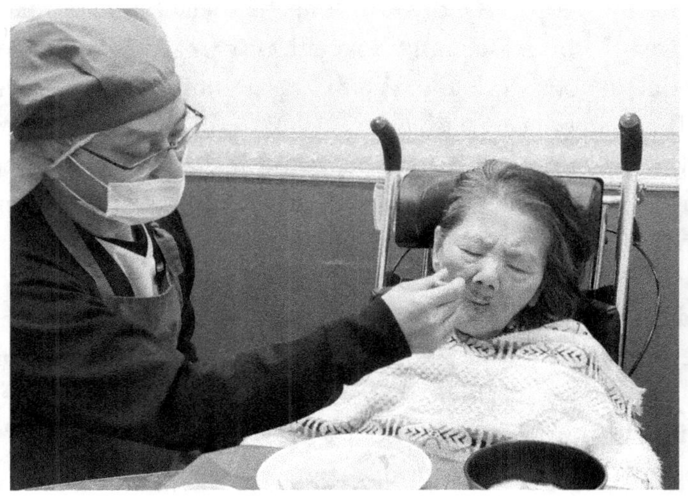

Mrs. Yamamoto's spark of vitality gives our caregivers vitality and energy.

Now, for professional caregivers: I encourage you to take pride in your work and have a vision for the future.

Compared to medical care, which is based on persuasive evidence, long-term care tends to be taken lightly. However, in the long-term care field, caregivers must tactfully respond on the spot to situations that cannot be measured by evidence, which I believe is a highly advanced ability that is different from other forms of medical care. Regardless of my title as chairman of an organization within the Housenka Group, I have the utmost respect for our caregivers who I am confident have this ability.

I do not want to sound like I am praising my own job, but I consider long-term care to be a noble profession where we can learn a lot from our seniors, including those with dementia. I also believe that long-term care is a challenging job that requires our full potential because it involves physical, intellectual, and emotional labor.

However, I also strongly believe that "challenging work" can lead to "great changes," and the more challenging the work, the more you will feel your growth. As the number of elderly people and people with dementia continues to increase, caregivers will be increasingly in demand and important. Hopefully, this will lead the social reputation and salary of caregivers to increase, and above all, to caregivers such as yourself taking pride in your work and discovering unlimited possibilities for the future. That is my sincere wish.

If even only one family member or professional caregiver currently engaging in dementia care feels that this book has given them a hint, made them feel better, or helped them see how to care for their loved one, that alone will make the publication worthwhile.

In dementia care we must continue to accumulate functional care methods that are not universal solutions. It is also a world that requires sensitivity. Sensitivity is not something that can be learned, but something we must refined on our own. The caregivers of Housenka, including myself, will also continue to steadily practice care and to refine our sensitivities in pursuit of better dementia care...

...to realize a dementia care paradise, where as many people as possible with dementia can live in peace.

ABOUT THE AUTHOR

Kenichi Akune, MA is currently serving as the Chairman of the social welfare corporation Fukusho Fukushikai, a part of Housenka Group in Japan. He has pursued a deep-rooted passion for dementia care, a calling profoundly influenced by his personal experiences during his teenage years. Akune witnessed his grandmother's battle with dementia, an ordeal that shaped not only his academic interests but also the course of his professional journey.

With a master's degree from Ryukoku University Graduate School of Sociology, specializing in Social Welfare, Akune has dedicated his career to serving the elderly. His expertise as a Certified Social Worker and Care Manager is complemented by a wealth of practical experience gained through various pivotal roles in the sector. He began his career working with different organizations before joining Housenka Group in 2002, coinciding with the opening of their specialized nursing home for the elderly.

Akune has held multiple leadership positions, including those of Facility Director and head of the administrative department. His leadership skills and dedication led to his appointment as Vice Chairman, and eventually, in 2017, he ascended to his current role as Chairman. Under his leadership, Housenka Group has continued to thrive, offering exemplary care and support to elders, and embodying the compassion that ignited Akune's initial foray into dementia care.

www.ingramcontent.com/pod-product-compliance
Lightning Source LLC
Chambersburg PA
CBHW070945260726
48661CB00003B/1134